TRIATHLETE MAGAZINE'S GUIDE TO FINISHING YOUR FIRST TRIATHLON

TRIATHLETE MAGAZINE'S GUIDE TO FINISHING YOUR FIRST TRIATHLON

T. J. Murphy

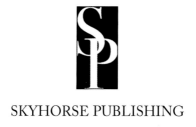

SKYHORSE PUBLISHING

Skyhorse Publishing books may be purchased in bulk at special discounts for sales promotion, corporate gifts, fund raising, or educational purposes. Special editions can also be created to specifications. For details, contact Special Sales Department, Skyhorse Publishing, 555 Eighth Avenue, Suite 903, New York, NY 10018 or info@skyhorsepublishing.com.

www.skyhorsepublishing.com

10 9 8 7 6 5 4 3 2 1

Library of Congress Cataloging-in-Publication Data

Murphy, T. J.
    Triathlete magazine's guide to finishing your first triathlon / by T. J. Murphy.
        p. cm.
    ISBN-13: 978-1-60239-234-2 (pbk. : alk. paper)
    ISBN-10: 1-60239-234-X (pbk. : alk. paper)
    1. Triathlon—Training. I. Triathlete. II. Title.
    GV1060.73.M87 2008
    796.42'57—dc22   2008000260

Printed in China

CONTENTS

ACKNOWLEDGMENTS

Thanks to Cam Elford, Rebecca Roozen, Jay Prasuhn, John Duke, Brad Culp, Matt Fitzgerald, and the rest of the staff at *Triathlete Magazine*. Special thanks to my editor for this book, Roy Wallack, coauthor of *Bike for Life: How to Ride to 100*. Roy's insight and expertise were invaluable to this book's completion.

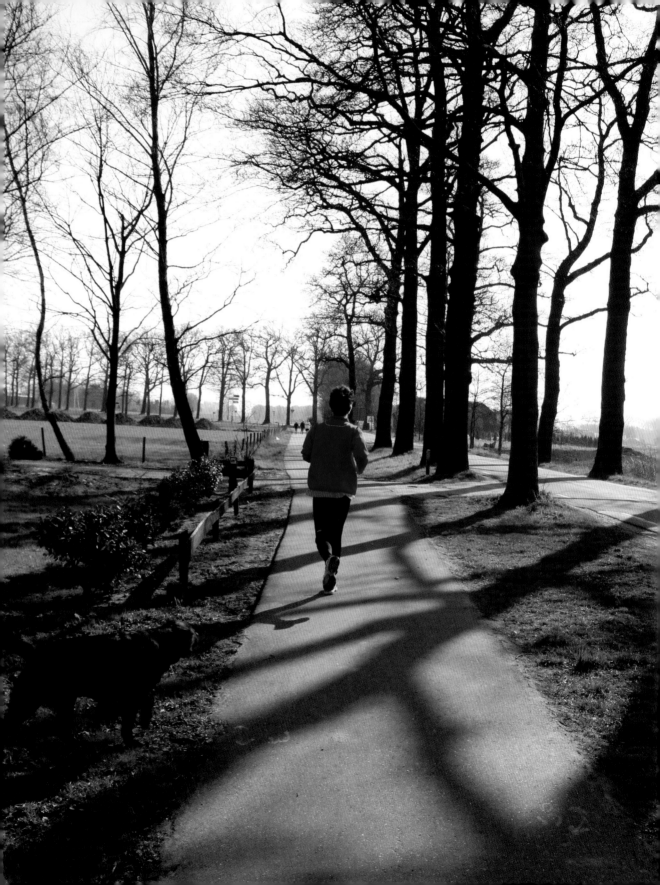

INTRODUCTION:
WHY YOU CAN BE
A TRIATHLETE

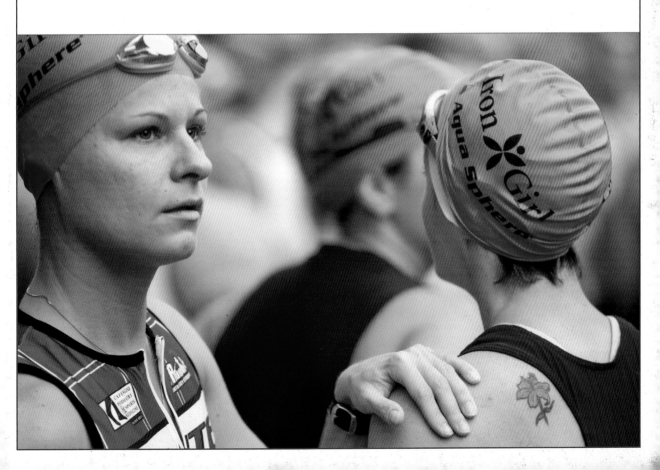

Here's the deal: You can be a triathlete. Whatever doubts you may harbor, whatever obstacles you face, whatever skepticism ignorant friends and loved ones spend toward you, *you can be a triathlete.*

I know this for a variety of reasons. For one thing, since I became a part of this sport 25 years ago—the last 12 of which I've been an editor for *Triathlete Magazine*—I've witnessed countless examples of people discovering the athlete within thanks to the fact they gave triathlon a try. Despite its image as the most demanding endurance sport in the world—one requiring participants to combine swimming, biking, and running—triathlon is a sport that welcomes all comers.

Are you out of shape? Are you fat? Have you tried and failed at dieting? When it comes to athletics, do you feel restricted to being a spectator? Triathlon wants you. Triathlon knows the truth: you can swim, bike, and run your way through a race and into the brother- and sisterhood of triathletes spread throughout the world.

Being a triathlete means embracing a healthy lifestyle. Being a triathlete means waking up in the morning feeling limber and powerful, energized and strong. It means watching less television

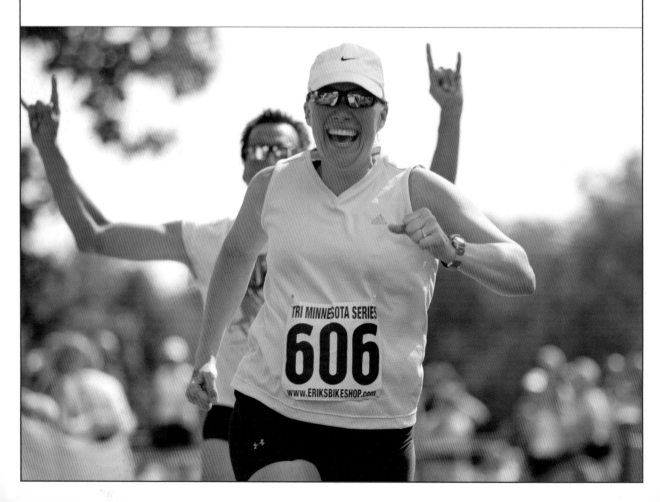

and getting in more workouts. It means setting goals for races, executing training plans and getting fit, completing the race and then going out for a celebratory post-race dinner.

Perhaps being overweight is a problem for you, one that anchors you to a depressing set of consequential actions. Diets are broken, followed by choices to numb you to reality: comfort foods, escaping into TV and alcohol, or worse. Fad diets are, for the most part, a moneymaking sham designed to sucker you into hopeful thinking and a credit card workout. Studies clearly indicate that dieting alone may help someone lose weight in the beginning, but after a year or so most everyone simply gains the weight back.

As you become a triathlete, your thinking will shift away from the nightmarish circle of wishing you could lose weight, of obsessing about calories and poor food choices. This is the trap that ensnares millions of Americans, one in which the focus is on feeling fat and down on yourself. It's a spiral of self-destruction.

You may be shackled by the belief that you are too fat, too old, too weak, or too untalented to become a triathlete. I know you're wrong. I've seen one young man, Chris Sustela, watch his weight tip the scale at over 300 pounds, prompting the decision to change. It took some

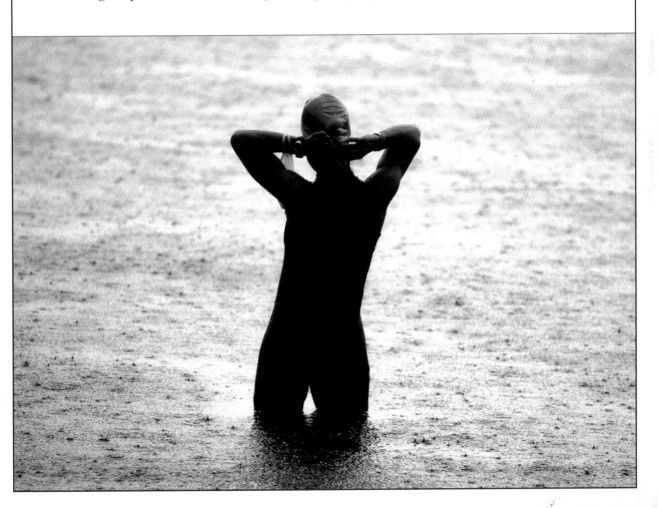

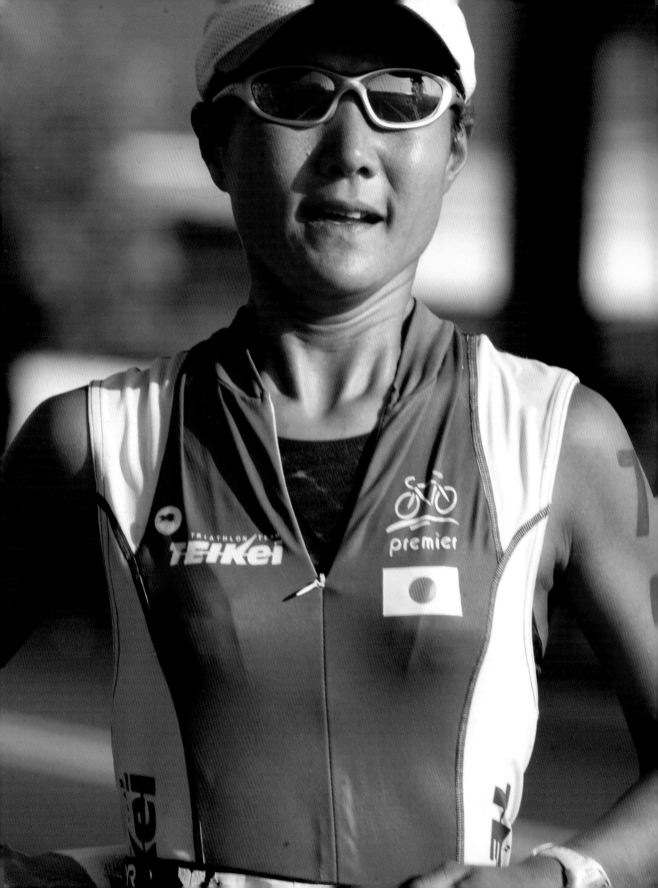

time, but within two years he was under 190 pounds and an Ironman triathlete. Recently I've borne witness to the birth of a new team of triathletes, Team Semper Fi, composed of U.S. Marines returning from Iraq missing either arms or legs or both. Team Semper Fi jumps into running races, marathons, and triathlons, completely rewriting the rules on what may have once limited a severely injured war veteran in life. I recently learned of a grade-school teacher who has completed several Ironmans, becoming a triathlete in the course of his recovery from clinical depression. Another growing movement within triathlon is Racing for Recovery, a group devoted to helping alcoholics and drug addicts sustain sober lives with the empowering benefits of being an athlete. Think you're too old to get into triathlon? Tell that to the 60- and 70-year-old men and women who are racing Ironmans (consisting of a 2.4-mile swim, 112-mile bike, and 26.2-mile run that can take up to seventeen hours to finish). I've seen this and much, much more over the last 25 years.

I know that your first step toward living life like an athlete—a life that is disciplined, energized, and fun—and becoming an athlete is in paving over the old thinking with a completely new layer of thought, standards, and self-expectations, followed immediately by small, easily performed action steps that slowly build upward. Next, an empowering momentum will take over. You will then complete your first triathlon, crossing the finish line and effectively putting a stake in the heart of the voice in your head that said, "I can't do it." Because you can—and just did.

This book is not a technical how-to guide for triathlon. We'll go through the basics, of course, but mostly this book is meant to show you, step-by-step and breath-for-breath, how to get started, get going, and finish your first triathlon with a smile on your face. We'll do that and the fitness will take care of itself—and guess what? In the process you'll learn the secret of how to stay fit the rest of your life: once you've become a triathlete, there's no turning back.

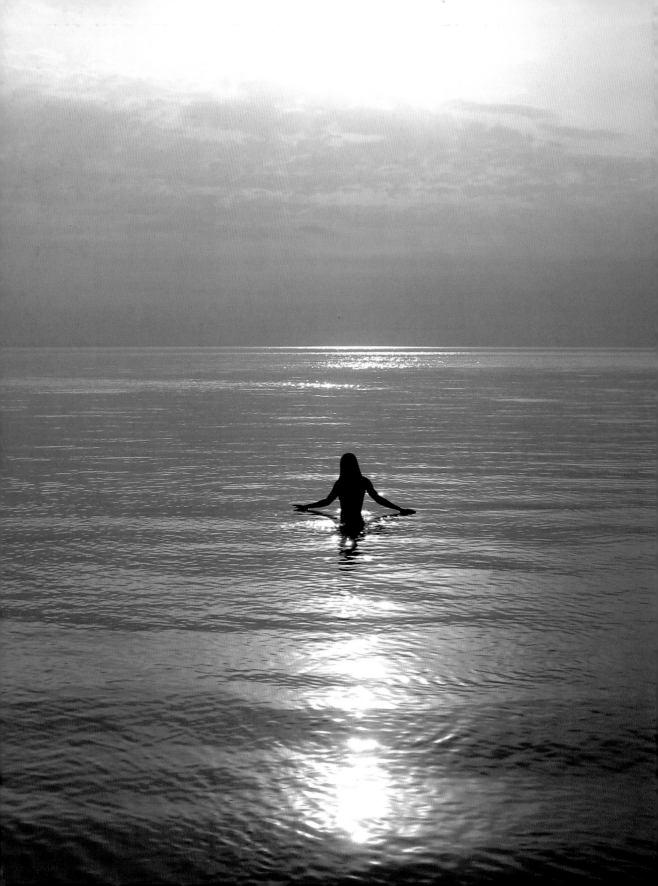

1

WHY TRIATHLON?

BECAUSE IT'S GOOD FOR YOU. AND IT'S FOR EVERYONE

It was in the early 1980s when I first became entranced by triathlon, having been one of the millions enthralled by images of the Hawaii Ironman. The race was broadcast on ABC's *Wide World of Sports*. The thought of an endurance race combining swimming, biking, and running was daunting and thrilling at the same time.

As triathlon grew over the next two decades, it developed an identity of being open to all. Triathlon became the place where limits were meant to be broken. No one was too old or untalented. The playing field wasn't restricted to elites. In fact, when you enter a triathlon, part of what makes the sport unique is that everyone, regardless of ability, rubs shoulders at the race venue. Triathlon has become a place that welcomes and encourages all. The physically challenged division in triathlon is symbolic of how the true heroes of the sport aren't always the elites in the front, but can be found in the stories within the pack and in the back of the pack.

The door is open to all who wish to participate. Choosing triathlon as your athletic passion is rich with benefits: it's fun, it's healthy, and it's a challenge that will revitalize your body and strengthen your mind.

The appeal of the swim-bike-run sport is broad. Here are a few of the reasons triathlon is an excellent pick for a lifelong sport:

1. Cross-training is built-in. Training for a triathlon requires a balanced exercise schedule. While swimming, biking, and running are all considered excellent activities to build up aerobic condition, they mix things up with regard to muscular conditioning. The muscles used across the three disciplines complement one another.
2. Triathlon builds a balanced physique. All the major muscle groups are put into play by the various activities in triathlon, resulting in a balanced musculature.
3. Triathlon strengthens the most important muscle: the heart. Studies clearly indicate that regular cardiovascular activity and a nutritious diet have numerous positive effects on heart health, longevity, and quality of life.
4. As compared to running-only exercise programs, you are less likely to sustain an overuse injury as a triathlete. Since swimming and cycling are nonimpact forms of training,

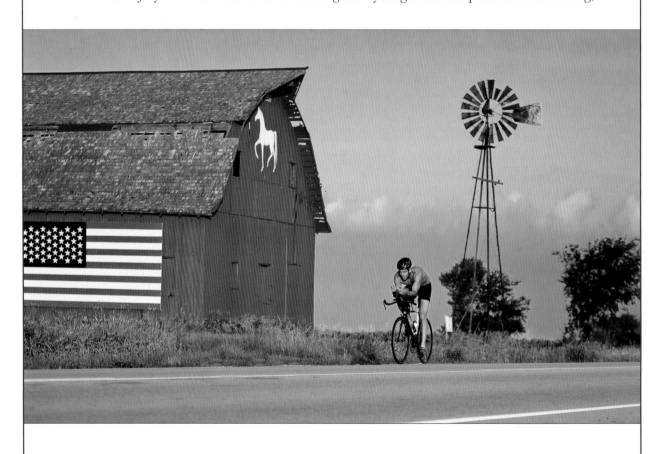

a triathlete spreads out the stress of running with active recovery days. In fact, many have been introduced to multisport because running injuries kept them on the sidelines.

5. The opportunities to race are diverse and plentiful. If you want to be a triathlete, you'll find ample races to choose from whether you live in California or Alabama. There are four primary race distances used in the American triathlon scene:

   a. Sprint-distance or "Tri-for-fun." Sprints are typically composed of the following: quarter-mile swim, 12-mile bike ride, and 3.1-mile run.

   b. Olympic-distance triathlons. This is a race replicating the actual event format used in the Olympics. It starts with a 1500-meter swim, continues with a 40-kilometer bike ride (25 miles), and finishes with a 10-kilometer (or 6.2-mile) run.

   c. Half Ironman. The half Ironman has been around a long time, but in recent years its popularity has become enormous, thanks in part to the new 70.3 Ironman series (70.3 signifying the total distance of the race). Half Ironmans begin with a 1.2-mile swim, transition to a 56.2-mile bike, and finish with a 13.1-mile run.

   d. Ironman. The full Ironman is the classic ultradistance event that helped put triathlon on the map after its creation in 1978. A 2.4-mile swim, 112-mile bike, and 26.2-mile run constitute this tremendous test of endurance and skill.

   e. XTERRA. The XTERRA race series is growing in popularity around the globe and has a rabid following. Considered an "all-terrain" event, XTERRAs are triathlons with mountain biking and trail running instead of cycling and running on roads.

6. Triathlons have become family events. When you start hunting for your first triathlon, you'll notice that many sprint races are part of triathlon festivals. If you want your kids to get in on it too, trifestivals typically have miniature triathlons for children. Also, if your spouse or partner is interested in running or walking a 5K, triathlon festivals often have these on the slate as well. The idea is to get everyone in on the action.

7. Parents wanting to set a good example of a fitness lifestyle for their kids can't do much better than triathlon. In today's culture, confronted by such a multitude of forces, from TV to video games to an automobile-based society, kids can easily get sucked into sedentary habits. Child obesity trends in the United States are

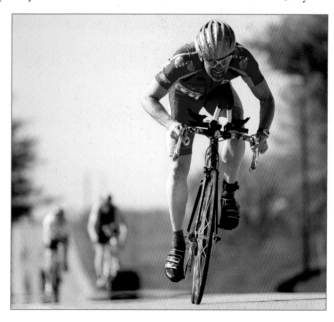

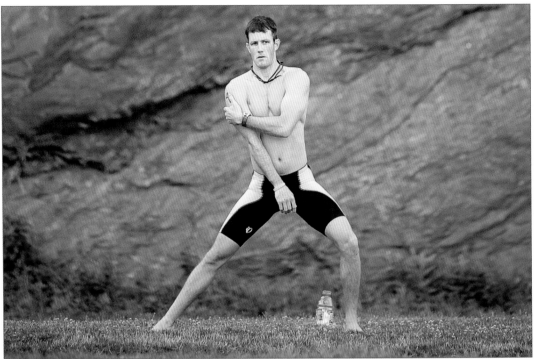

startling, giving rise to a deadly increase in the number of childhood cases of diabetes. Parents who buck these trends are likely to inspire their children to follow suit.

To get you started, let's discuss the core principles of how to transform yourself into a competitive triathlete.

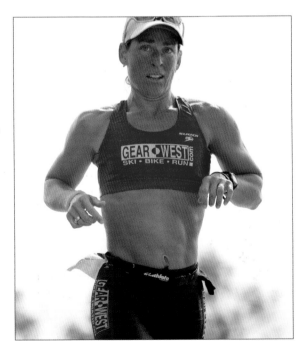

2
THE
DECISION

EMBRACING THE CHALLENGE, THE CAMARADERIE, THE FUN

Okay, so you like the idea of being a triathlete. It may be nothing more profound than wanting to have a triathlete body. If you worry that this is a shallow desire, don't despair. While a handful of triathletes may have migrated into multisport to chase Olympic medals or glory on the Ironman racecourse, I'm willing to bet that a Zogby Poll would show that more than 90 percent of the people participating in triathlon got into it because of what is produced when you expose the human body to consistent swimming, biking, running, and nutrition: a triathlete.

Whatever the initial impulse, other benefits await. For one thing, it feels good. If you've been stuck in a cycle of self-abuse governed by a desire for junk food and couch time, the feeling waiting for you after as little as a week of living like an athlete is too remarkable to be accurately described.

Triathlon is a competitive sport. For the most part, it's a sport of competition with the self. For many, the goal is to finish. If you've ever watched a triathlon in person, you will likely have noticed a deep camaraderie existing within the field of triathletes. They're all in it together. They cheer each other on and help each other out. It's not uncommon to see friendships emerge between racers who have endured the long middle miles of the last leg of the event, the run.

Perhaps you consider yourself a noncompetitive person. If so, I want you to visit this notion and consider revising it. We respond naturally to challenge. It's invigorating. Setting a competitive goal (just finishing a first triathlon is a terrific initial goal) immediately gets the blood pumping. You'll choose a race several months off in the distance, fill out the application, and send in your money. Once you've committed yourself to a race—and I'll encourage you to tell others who will be supportive of your goal—you will receive an adrenaline-producing burst of urgency. We are goal-oriented creatures, and the commitment to a goal conducts an inner source of energy that will be exceptionally helpful in nudging the worst of couch potatoes out of a TV-induced rut.

Don't fear competition. Embrace it. It's fun; trust me. There may be a tinge of fear connected to the idea of competing. Good. Don't worry, you're not going to be in a one-on-one Olympic final swimming against Michael Phelps. We'd all get our ass kicked. Rather, you're going to be competing against yourself. This is the competitor you'll be taking on: any side of your personality preferring comfort and numbness to living the athletic life. Like I said in the introduction, once you've defeated this first foe, there is no going back.

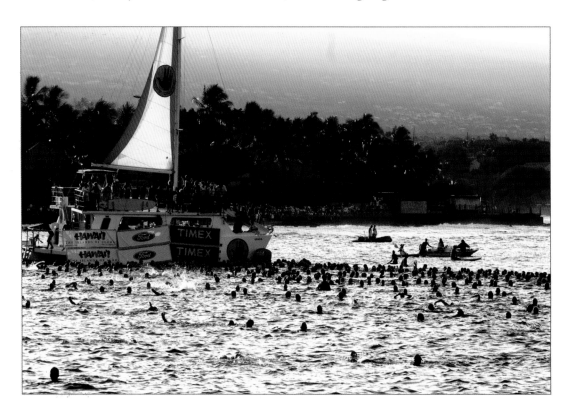

Years ago Nike put together an ad that, in a way, illustrated this competition. It was a print magazine ad, a photograph of a robust businessman in a restaurant. From the image of the man, you figured he was wealthy and had a decent expense account. It looked like he'd just finished a feast of a dinner, and was now enjoying a glass of brandy and a cigar—all the finest in terms of the creature comforts our society dogs us with. In the image, as the man gazed out the window, it was a stormy night, miserable out, cold and wet, and the businessman was insulated from it within the warm glow of the restaurant. But as he was looking out into the night, a runner was bounding past the window, into the wind and rain, on a training run.

I loved the ad. With a single photograph, Nike told the underlying story between the two choices: The businessman was doing his best to insulate himself from any sort of discomfort and pain. The food may have tasted good, but it was a fleeting joy. The brandy may provide a jolt of inebriation—also fleeting, and it comes with the damaging cost drugs exact. The runner was burning his way through discomfort, and as any endurance athlete knows, there's no better feeling in the world then working out or just having finished a workout. We all have days where it's a little tough to get out the door, but once we do, we're glad we did. This is another secret of triathletes: Although you may feel tired, anguished, stressed, and don't want to go to the gym or get on the bike, you have faith that once you do, you'll be relieved you did.

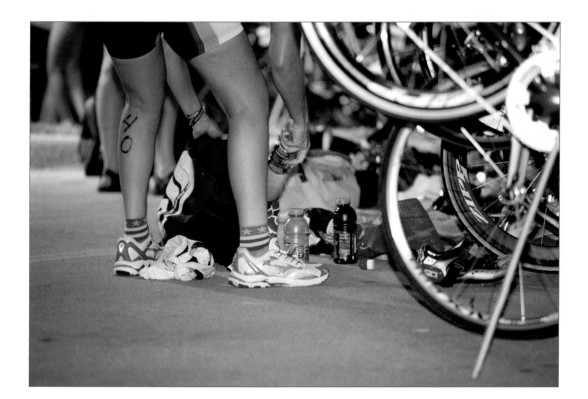

This leads us to the first new belief I want you to subscribe to: Exercise is not painful. Exercise feels good. Exercise is an ultimate in self-indulgence.

Your first step in becoming a triathlete is this: to decide you are a triathlete and to realize that within you is an athlete waiting to be realized. Once you make this decision, your mind will find comfort in the process of living the life the way an athlete lives life: You'll become protective of the hour you need here and there throughout the week to train, you will begin to accumulate tastes for healthier power foods and meals that will enhance your training and recovery from training. You'll feel increasingly healthier and stronger, with more energy, better sleep, and greater self-confidence. You'll soon get the sensory payoff from these actions: it feels good and you'll want more. There will be no turning back.

It starts off with the decision to do it. To know that within you is an athlete and that you will that enjoy the small, incremental step-by-step process entailed in the remainder of this book is an empowering moment in anyone's life. I will ask you to start small, be consistent, to enjoy it, and we'll slowly build our way up.

As Brian Walton, the internationally respected head coach of Cadence Cycling and Multi-sport, says, the first weeks of training are all about giving the athlete a taste of the positive "drug" training serves up. "After I get them hooked, the rest is easy."

As a man thinketh, so in his heart is he. —Proverbs 23:7

Today is the day you decide you're a triathlete. Write it down in a diary, carve it into the wall, dig it into the dirt. Chuck the past, don't worry about the present, and let's get started.

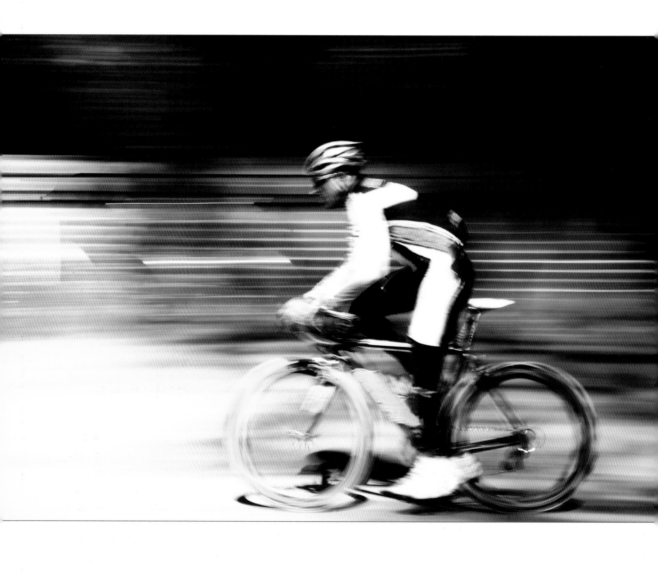

3
THE BIG PICTURE

AN 18-WEEK GAME PLAN, FROM YOUR FIRST ATHLETIC STEPS TO TRIATHLON RACE DAY

Terry Laughlin is the head coach of Total Immersion Swimming. Laughlin has authored books, written countless articles for national magazines, and produced videos for anyone and everyone who wants to become a good swimmer. Laughlin also leads two-day workshops around the country, and in a weekend he routinely guides people away from the worst of swim strokes into a clean, relaxed, and efficient swimming style. I can report accurately on this because I am one such case.

Like many people new to triathlon, when I got into the sport, the swim leg was my biggest concern. I knew I was terrible. Swim technique is burned into your brain, a neurological pattern. I would go to swim classes and swim team workouts, and inevitably the coach would see me catastrophically splashing my way, slowly, through lap after lap, and then give me a list of things to change. Do this with your legs, this with your elbows, do this with your hands, breathe like this, shape your stroke like this, rotate your trunk like this. I would obediently nod throughout the lecture and try and correct everything on the long list of tweaks. I would have a lightning storm in my brain, shorting everything out, and I was sure little had changed because the next time the coach saw me, I could see the look in his eye: *This guy's pathetic.*

My experience with Laughlin was the polar opposite. Laughlin has a warm presence, and speaks with the calm assurance of a Jedi master. As opposed to the stereotypical swim coach who demands lung-searing cardiovascular efforts, Laughlin urges you to relax and take it easy. He doesn't simply ask you to jump in the pool and start swimming as he issues you Band-Aids for your stroke. In the two-day workshop I attended, Laughlin started us out with the simplest of movements in the water. He would ask us to practice these movements over and over, cautioning us against anything resembling struggle. Each drill was a single, specific, and easy to accomplish movement in the water. We would practice each one in a relaxed manner, moving easily through the pool, and Laughlin and his coaches would watch and talk us through it. After hours of practicing the movements, none of it mentally or physically tiring, Laughlin revealed to us that what we were doing—the final combination of simple movements—was our new swimming stroke. We all

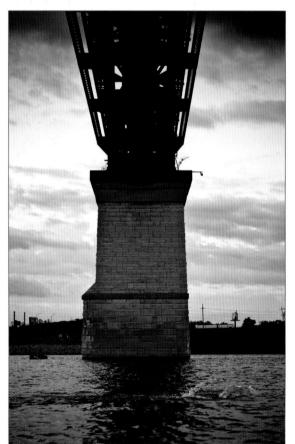

looked at each other, sharing the epiphany. My previous experiences with swim coaches trying to teach me how to fix my stroke were nothing short of torture. Laughlin's method can be accurately described as a meditation. It was free of frustration and stress. We'd leave the workshop at the end of the day in a state of bliss.

Laughlin refers to his approach as "Avoiding struggle." In his book, *Triathlon Swimming Made Easy*, he explains the process. Laughlin believes the exceptional improvement made by students in his two-day workshops is due to "muscle amnesia" and "martial-arts swimming." He writes, "By teaching with movements their nervous systems don't recognize as swimming, we've given them 'muscle amnesia,' a blank slate for learning new skills and bypassing old habits."

I'm mentioning all of this for two reasons. One, I heartily recommend you seek out a Laughlin workshop, particularly if you worry about the swim leg of triathlon. The books and tapes are a worthwhile substitution or an excellent addition.

Secondly, and more to the point of this chapter, it's my wish that your entry into triathlon resemble this approach. For some, the thought of being a triathlete and racing a triathlon conjures up extraordinary images of super athletes and intimidating situations. Rather, the approach offered in this book seeks to channel the subtle and calming experience of a Total Immersion swim workshop: with a slow, steady rhythm, we will start with small, brief, and easy to accomplish tasks that easily stack on top of each other. There will be no hurling you into an epic ocean swim or onto a ride up a mountain or an interval track workout. We are not going to cut your diet down to 1,000 calories a day and have you take up a nonfat vegan diet.

THE 18-WEEK GAME PLAN

I assume that right now you have little or no momentum when it comes to eating right and exercising. That's fine. If you're someone who is exercising a lot and eating a nutritious diet, this book is probably best passed on to a friend or loved one whom you've inspired to embrace an athletic lifestyle.

Working within a sequence of incremental steps, you will first undergo a six-week "Basic Training" boot camp that will phase you painlessly into a healthy, athletic lifestyle. That will be followed by a systematic 12-week program that will make you a triathlete and leave you at a peak for your first race. It's 18 weeks from non-athlete to triathlete, a step-by-step journey of discovery that will have you mastering a set of simple, basic habits and building upon them. Here are the accomplishments you'll chalk up in the next four months:

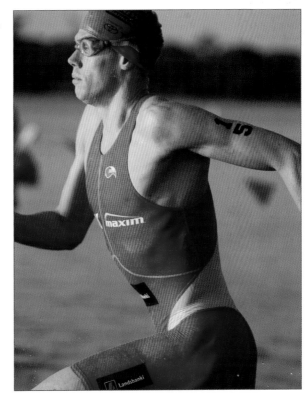

1. **Decide to be an athlete:** You made the decision at the end of the last chapter to go for an active, athletic lifestyle. You will build a foundation on top of this new self-concept.
2. **Get medical clearance:** An essential step of any exercise program is getting your physician's okay to embark on a new health and fitness program. In addition to a thorough checkup, an important topic to discuss with your doctor is your medical history specific to your heart.

3. **The six-week "intro to fitness" makeover:** A new athletic life starts with simple steps. You won't become a full-blown triathlete in six weeks, the length of the introductory phase you will read about in chapter 6. In fact, you shouldn't even try. Your body and mind is not yet ready for the rigors of real training. Nothing is more shocking, mentally and physically, than jumping into a cold pool of water—in this case, a wholesale makeover of lifelong habits. To minimize the shock of thinking and acting like a triathlete, you are going to stick your toe in the water first, then slowly acclimate. Six weeks does not sound like a long time, but studies show that you can affect profound differences in lifestyle habits and attitudes in that span. You will tippy-toe into two changes simultaneously: diet and exercise.

4. **Rethink your diet:** Food = fuel. Don't think "food"—think "rocket fuel." From now on, you are eating certain foods not to lose weight (believe me, that will come natu-

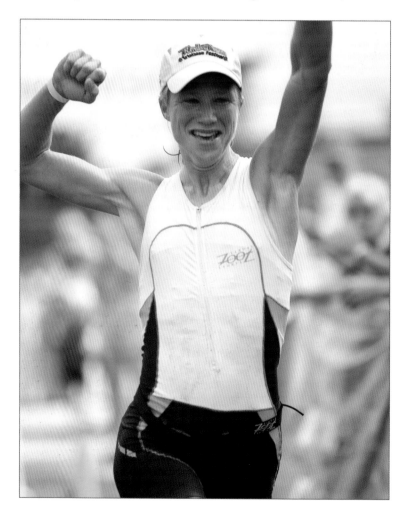

rally), but purely for energy, to put gasoline in the tank. Over a six-week period, our intention will be to incorporate a diet plan that provides your increasingly exercise-modified, high-performance body with an appropriate high-performance source of energy. The fact that this "fuel" happens to be very healthy is a side benefit. Every week we will add something to your diet, and explain the nutritional principle behind it.

5. **Get your body moving:** As you transform food into fuel, you will also build the habit of taking time, in the form of a ritual of performing simple, low-key aerobic exercise. If you have not been particularly athletic, this may be as simple as a walk or scenic bike ride, but the idea is to ingrain the idea of daily exercise and the enjoyment of it. By putting your body to work, you will be laying a new, habitual pattern over old behaviors. As you progress, this workout will become more specific and more valuable in preparing your

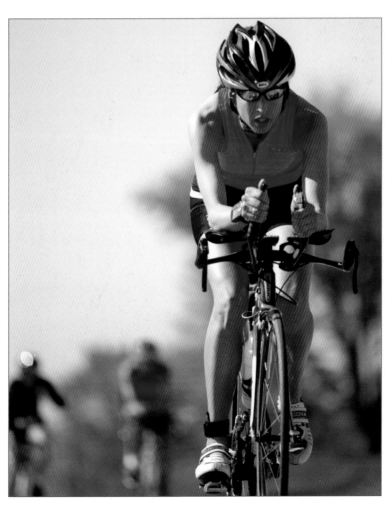

body for triathlon training. Once this sinks in, you'll guard this time with zealousness. You may have a job, family responsibilities, and serve on the PTA board, but this time is yours and you will let no one interfere.

6. **Write it down:** Every day, so you don't forget what you have done, you'll write it all down. You will also build the habit of keeping a logbook. A logbook offers a galvanizing power to the athlete. The recording of your daily diet and exercise accomplishments will energize and focus your daily efforts. As an athlete, this diary will serve as a source of motivation and accountability, and as evidence of your efforts.

7. **Pick a race:** This is the fun part. Upon completion of the initial six-week "intro to fitness" phase, you will select your target. You will choose an appropriate race and submit an entry. It's now time to begin real triathlon training.

8. **Initiate your training program:** With a race goal in mind, you will spend the next 12 weeks training to complete it. The training will be fun, feel good, and slowly, gently prepare you for the event.

9. **The race:** As you'll discover, race day is the icing on the cake. This is where you congregate with other triathletes and put it all on the line. This is where you test yourself. This is where you celebrate.

10. **Now, dream big. Real big:** Part of your reward for completing your first triathlon is plotting what's next. Being a triathlete means training for the love of it. But now is the time to take things up a notch. After your first triathlon, it's time to think big. Whatever goal you set: finishing an Olympic-distance triathlon, a half Ironman, or Ironman triathlon, it's within your reach. Now that you're a triathlete, it's a matter of planning, time, and execution.

Throughout the entire process this book seeks to provide you with a basic education in the principles of training, what's what with equipment, and the essential vocabulary of triathlon. We will break down and demystify what at first glance is a complex sport. And as we do, you will break down your own barriers. Stick with it, and there is only one guarantee: in 18 weeks, you will be a new person.

4

SHOPPING SPREE

**HALF THE FUN OF TRIATHLON IS ACQUIRING NEW GEAR.
AND THIS SPORT HAS A LOT OF IT**

Bikes. Wet suits. Running shoes. Goggles. Tubes. Aerobars. Energy gels. My god—where does it end?

Yes, triathlon is a shopper's delight. Oodles of gear to ogle over, most of it actually useful for comfort, safety, and shaving valuable seconds and minutes off your time. But thankfully, I will tell you that you honestly don't need most of it at the beginning, when finishing is the real issue and a few seconds here and there is meaningless. This chapter will teach you what you need and help you limit the damage to your bank account. After all, you have enough stress already without having to worry about making the house payment.

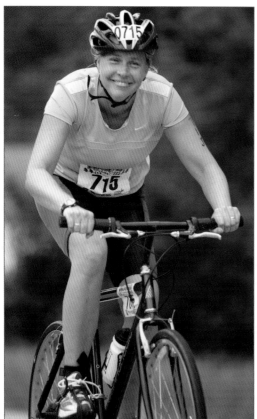

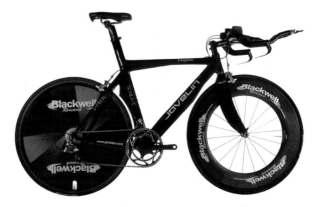

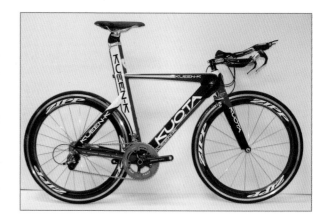

CYCLING GEAR

When you're talking about triathlon gear, the first issue that almost always arises is the bike—and I don't mean riding it. Bicycles themselves are complex, mechanical, and utterly frightening to many first timers. And going into a bike shop doesn't help. Many people step out of bike shops completely intimidated.

Well, take it easy. I maintain that for a first triathlon, just about any bike you have handy will do the job. I've been witness to dozens of triathlons over the years, and I've seen many first-time triathletes get through the bike portion of the race on cheapo mountain bikes or geeky commuter bikes. Sure, they'd don't deliver the jaw-dropping power-image of a $7,000 Cervélo time trial bike, but even if you have money burning holes through your pockets, I wouldn't recommend to any beginning triathlete to buy a time trial bike.

If you want to buy a bike for your first years in the sport of triathlon, my suggestion is to buy a good road bike. Why not a tri bike or time trial bike? Because despite the sleek, rocket-like look of a tri bike, you still have to pedal it to make it go anywhere. And here's the deal with aerodynamics and a tri bike: First, unless you're going pretty fast, you really don't acquire much in aerodynamic savings. When you start closing in or surpassing an average of 20 mph in a race, then it's probably time to consider a tri bike. Second, to net aerodynamic value on a tri bike, you have to ride in the aero position, meaning your arms and elbows are set into the tri bars and stay there for long periods of time. I can't tell you how many times I've been at longer triathlons where I've watched triathletes who have probably been in the sport a fair amount of time riding expensive, tricked out tri bikes, and they're so uncomfortable riding in an aerodynamic position that they're sitting bolt upright, hands on the bars and head high in the air. The bike might as well be a mountain bike when you ride this way.

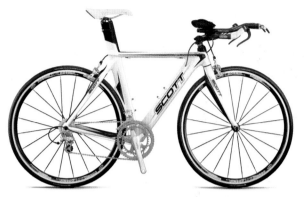

One of the key differences between a road bike and a tri bike is the geometry of the frame. Tri bikes have what is known as an "aggressive" geometry, designed to help configure your body into a more aerodynamic shape. With a good fitting session and strong set of core muscles, this shape and position can indeed be fairly comfortable. But in general it's best to first cultivate a love of cycling, and more often than not this won't happen if your initial bike is a tri bike.

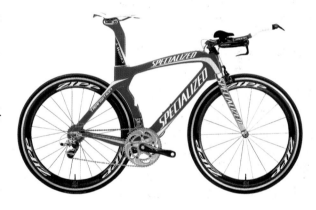

Road bikes on the other hand *can* cultivate this love affair with zero emission traveling. If you have the money and the desire to invest in a good road bike (I suggest having at least $1,000 to spend), then fantastic. Buying your first training/racing bike is a special experience and will bolster your commitment to the sport.

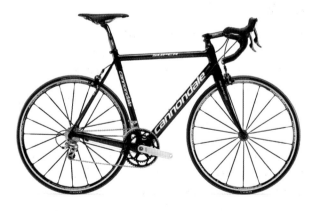

Where should you buy your first bike? If you live in a city, it's likely you have several options in the way of bike shops. I advise committing yourself to visiting them all before you plop down the credit card. For one thing, rarely does one bike shop have a complete collection of models to choose from, and, more importantly, I think it's a good idea to scope them all out and consider establishing a relationship with the shop that "feels" best to you.

There are two ingredients that are most important to making a successful bike purchase:

1. **Fit:** The bike needs to be the right size and fit correctly to your body. This is where a knowledgable staff at your bike shop can really help you. The best salesperson will be aggressive in making sure you're comfortable and fit well on the bike.
2. **Look:** The bike must appeal to you. In other words, you should dig your bike. It's your race car. You should look at it and feel your pulse rate speed up. As Multisports.com coach Paul Huddle suggests, if you think a bike makes for a bitchin' ride, it will be a bitchin' ride.

When you do test ride a bike, pay particular attention to how smoothly it shifts gears. You want a fairly seamless operation. Ask what the store's policy is on tune-ups in the first weeks and months of owning the bike. Look for a fairly liberal one.

More bike stuff: Keep the credit card handy.

Okay, buying a bike is one thing, but it doesn't end there.

Pedals: Today is the age of the clipless pedal, and as unnatural as they may seem at first, it's best to throw yourself into the learning curve. Before you know it, you won't even be thinking about them. But at first, it's a good idea practicing clipping and unclipping from your pedals on a quiet road or in a huge, empty parking lot. Downtown New York City is not the place to get the hang of these.

Shoes: Bike shoes are an important purchase. Shoes are cut differently, and I've found that making sure the width is appropriate to your foot is key. If the shoe is too narrow, it can feel as though it's cutting off the blood flow in the foot. If it's too wide, you feel as if you're sliding around all over the place inside the shoe, a precursor to blisters. I know many triathletes who don't wear socks with their bike shoes, but this is not a practice I'd suggest for first-timers. Good cycling socks will help make the sport more enjoyable for you.

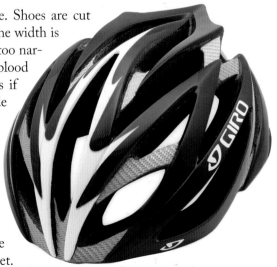

Helmet: You have three primary concerns. First, it needs to be certified for safety by the CPSC, a sticker that you'll see inside the helmet.

Second, it needs to fit snugly on your head, snugly enough that if you fall it will protect you. Finally, it needs to be comfortable. Buy a helmet that is relatively lightweight and vented; this will increase the comfort in warmer conditions.

Tools: A set of Allen keys is essential for simple adjustments like tightening up certain bolts or moving the seat. You'll also need a set of tire irons and extra tubes for when you need to repair a flat.

Clothing: A pair of bike shorts and a cycling jersey, with pockets, will do wonders for your overall comfort level when riding. Sunglasses will protect you from dust and debris that can hit your eyes.

Cycling gloves: Not a necessity, but they again add to your general comfort on a longer ride.

RUNNING SHOES

Running shoes may be the single most important piece of equipment when it comes to preventing overuse injury. Running incurs a repetitive impact stress that is channeled through the foot. When the foot strikes the pavement, it turns in a way that is called pronation. How the foot pronates, underpronates, or overpronates can send stresses through the rest of your skeletal system and, particularly if you're not yet adapted to running, can cause annoying pains in the calves, shins, knees, hips, and back. If you have a high arch, for example, one common ailment running can produce is chronic arch pain, also known as plantar fasciitis.

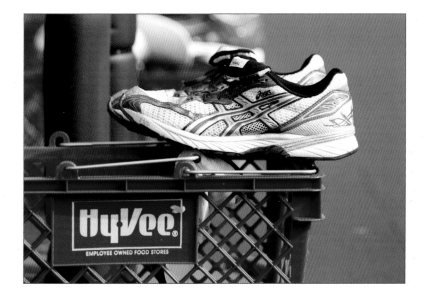

The best defense against overuse injuries in running is first and foremost using a gradual approach to the activity. While your cardiovascular system can improve quite quickly, followed by the muscles, tendons and ligaments need more time to increase in strength. They will always need your attention as you sink yourself into the endurance world. Stretching is especially important if you're a bit older.

Running shoes can do a lot to aid this prevention effort. If you're worried about running injuries right off the bat because you've had problems with your feet or your knees, there are simple tests to try and identify what kind of biomechanics you tend toward. However, a footstrike and gait analysis performed at a good running podiatrist is usually the best way to determine all of the idiosyncracies of your feet.

When buying running shoes, you don't only want to try and match the width of your foot, but the shape of it. Running shoes mostly come in a semi-curved shape, but there are models that are straight-lasted and curve-lasted. At a running shoe store, ask the salesman to help you identify what models of shoes might be good to try on.

Expect to spend upwards of $60 on your running shoes. Anything cheaper is usually worthless and will leave you prone to trouble. Lightweight shoes can certainly feel dreamy in the store, but you're going to get a longer cushioning life out of your shoes if they have some beef to them. Shoes weighing between 12 and 14 ounces are the way to go. If the shoe is under ten ounces, leave it alone until you've transformed yourself into a 120-pound Kenyan.

When trying shoes on, it's best to do so later in the day or after a run. You want to fit your foot when it's more swollen so that you don't accidentally buy a size that's too small and ultimately bangs up against your toes. Leaving a bit of space in the toe box is generally a good rule of thumb.

One of the most important questions you'll find yourself asking is, "How often should I buy new running shoes?" This is a tough one. Running shoes can break down a lot faster than you'd think they should (they're not cheap). And when they've broken down, you can feel the increase in impact stress when running on the pavement. For this reason alone, only use your running shoes for your walking and running workouts. Don't wear them around the house, in the yard, or off to run errands. Every step you take in them will add to shortening their lifespan. If you can afford to, I recommend replacing running shoes about every three months or five hundred miles of running, whichever comes first. If you have the bucks to change shoes earlier, it's a good investment.

Here are several additional tips on running shoes:

1. **Size doesn't matter:** Don't rely on what size work shoes you might wear when you go to try on shoes. In fact, throw this number out the window. Running shoes tend to run differently than other shoes, and as a matter of fact, I've seen shoes within the same brand run a half size off of each other. So by all means get measured by the sales staff if you want, but be prepared to judge each shoe by the way it wraps around your heel and embraces your forefoot.

2. **Test 'em:** This may mean running around the store or outside of it, but getting a chance to see how the shoes feel to run in is exceptionally valuable information. Some running

shoe stores even have treadmills that you can use, and in a perfect world they have a podiatrist there who can evaluate your footstrike and gait.

3. **Up-front shock absorber:** Most running shoe companies do an impressive job with this these days. Back in the 1980s, the forefoots of shoes seemed to be an afterthought and were prone to early breakdown. Still, ask if the shoe has an air sole or gel in the forefoot. This can help lengthen the cushioning life of the shoe.

4. **Think long-term:** Huge superstores have marginalized many of the "technical" running shoe stores that flourished in the 1980s and 1990s, but in big cities you can usually find a true running shoe store. These hangouts are often staffed by runners and can be a great source of expertise and advice.

5. **Arch support:** Most running shoes have little in the way of arch support. Several generic orthotics are on the market that can add a lot to your running shoes in the form of basic arch protection and rearfoot control.

Shoe talk. Here are the basics when it comes to the general types of running shoes available:

Stability shoes: Stability shoes are designed to prevent you from overpronating.

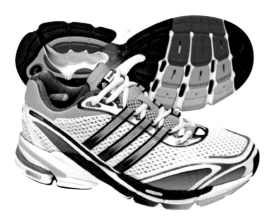 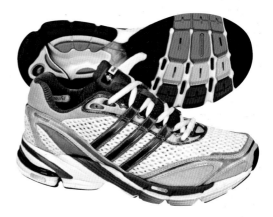

Cushion shoes: Cushion shoes, like the Nike Air Max, are designed to give you maximum protection from impact shock.

Motion control shoes: Motion control shoes are usually heavy duty trainers that are built on a wide last and designed for ultimate protection.

Lightweight trainers: Lightweight trainers are usually 11 ounces or less in a men's size nine, and are best used by experienced distance runners/triathletes who want a faster shoe for speed training. They also work well as a race shoe.

Trail shoes: Trail shoes are built with rugged outsoles and tough upper materials to allow you to thrash them on technical trails.

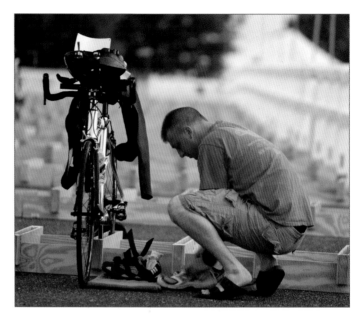

Like in buying a bicycle, treat the occasion of buying new running shoes with a celebratory attitude. New equipment signifies launching into new training. Enjoy the moment!

SWIMMING GEAR

Thankfully, swim gear is relatively simple. Mostly what you'll need outside a swimsuit is a pair of goggles. Again, like shoes and bikes, fit is king when it comes to goggles. Here are some general guidelines to getting set up with goggles:

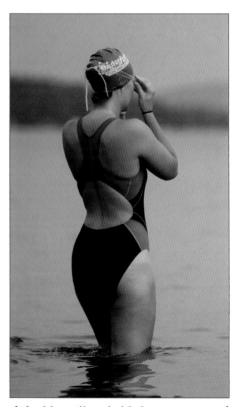

1. **Fit is everything:** Goggles that don't leak are going to mean the world to you. Believe me. I've had more trouble with this than anyone (at least it seems like that). Once you find a pair that fits you well, stock up in case you lose or break the pair you're using. Store the backups in a special location.
2. **Tint:** If you're going to be swimming in an outdoor pool, you should buy tinted googles. There's nothing like turning for air and getting an eyeful of retina-singeing sunshine.
3. **Anti-fog:** Sounds gross, but a bit of spit smeared on your goggles is a simple defense against fogging. Fogging is right up there with leaking in terms of driving you nuts. Anti-fog drops are also available to help you deal with this problem.

Other items: If you start working with a coach or masters program, you'll become acquainted with various tools at the poolside. Kickboards, paddles, floats, and the like will probably be incorporated

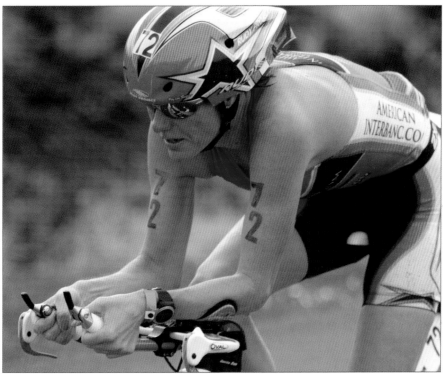

into your game. The one item you might want whether you work with a coach or go to the pool solo is a set of long fins. Long fins will help you build your kick strength up and also give you some locomotion to practice drills with.

BIG-GUY BIKES

Support your Clydesdale Power with the right equipment

Being a "Clydesdale"—triathlonese for having a big, heavy body—has its benefits and advantages. One benefit is that many races give you your own category, so you are officially competing against other triathletes who weigh over 200 pounds, not the tiny Lilliputians you see in all the magazines. One drawback, of course, is that moving that big, heavy body presents a challenge because it requires a lot more effort, which is what led to the creation of the category in the first place.

The challenge of moving that mass especially comes to a head on climbs. That uphill disadvantage can be verified mathematically. After all, triathlon is a sport that matches your strength (the watts you produce) and your lung capacity (VO_2). Since VO_2 is a measurement of your oxygen consumption per kilogram of body weight, you are automatically at a disadvantage when it comes to going up.

Does this mean you won't ever win?

"Absolutely not!" says Greg Bourque, a San Diego acupuncturist who is the rider/ director of the Team Seasilver professional cycling team (www.AlternativeEdge.net). "But you do need to make the appropriate equipment and attitude adjustments to put all the variables in your favor." He says that Clydesdales can sabotage themselves into under-performing by being sidelined or slowed by poor equipment choices.

"You know the old phrase, 'A poor worker blames his tools'? It's often true in triathlon—especially on race day for some reason," says Bourque. "How often have you heard, 'I could've of won if I didn't break my $#@% thing!' The reality is that you need to accommodate for your size and the big-time power that goes with it."

Bourque, a Clydesdale himself, has first-hand knowledge of the big-boy issue. "I can't help but hear the mantra of my first coach when I flatted out of the Nova Scotia Team Time Trial Championships in '84. 'THE TIME FOR EXCUSES HAS PASSED!' he told me. Needless to say I didn't go to Nationals that year."

Here's Borque's analysis of your big-guy bike from top to bottom.

Saddle

The whole point of a saddle is to support your *sitting bones,* so if your derriere is on the wide side then you need a wide saddle. It is that simple. Saddles with a hollow seat rail should be avoided, as they can break. Also, don't scrimp on comfort. Choose the saddle that most feels like the living room sofa—not necessarily the most expensive saddle on the market.

Frame

Firstly, get a bike that fits. If you close your eyes and it feels right then away you go. For athletes who require a large size, forget about the traditional diamond frame and get an XXL compact frame. The reason being that your center of gravity is already too high, and if you want to corner and descend like Floyd Landis you need to drop your center of gravity as low as possible. As far as frame materials, Bourque has broken them all—steel, aluminum, carbon, and scandium. "There isn't any reliability in frame materials," says Bourque. "The best you can do is not use a first-year product. Let those frames get tested by the pro teams for a year and see if they are still selling them the next year."

Handlebars and Stem

This is not the place to sacrifice integrity for weight. "I have seen far too many days ruined with snapped lightweight stem bolts and outright material failure," says Bourque.

A side note on clip-on aero bars: if you have etched or crimped your bars installing them, then you must throw your bars in the trash. "Sadly, I learned this lesson the hard way going into turn three of the Pomona Valley Stage Race," says Bourque. "It was the last stage with only two of 50 laps to go when I ended up having a handlebar in each hand and the pavement rushing toward my face. These were new bars but I overtightened the clip-on bolts and lost some weight the hard way—by leaving it on the ground. I would also advise against buying used bars—they straighten easily after a fall but will never be the same."

Wheels and Tires

Obviously, you can spend a lot on wheels and mostly get what you pay for. The fewer spokes you have, the more messed up the wheel will be after you clock a pothole. The narrower the hub, the less lateral stability the wheel will have. If you break more than three spokes on the same wheel then chances are it's toast and you need to rebuild it with a new rim. If you think you need the lightest wheel out there, then you just need to watch the Tour de France and you will see guys driving the break riding on box rims that probably cost $60 a pair from Taiwan. When it comes to tires, you have only one option—ride a 23c tire size. If you ride a 20c or 19c then you will flat before you make it to the start. 23c-width tires are just as fast and puncture far less. "I do stress that you suck it up and put on new tires before the race if you don't have separate training and race wheels," says Bourque.

Bicycle and Mind

"Finally," says Bourque. "let us not forget the final component to a complete package—your mind. If you believe that you are at a disadvantage because of your weight then you've already lost."

"Cycling is a beautiful sport because athletes of all shapes and sizes can be competitive," he says. "Where one individual might have a high VO_2, and the other a massive wattage, the winner will be the one who simply knows how to commit and suffer until he turns inside out and blood spurts from his eyes."

Bourque likes to point to superstar Clydesdale cyclist Magnus Backstedt, a relatively massive 210-pounder who has won the grueling Paris–Roubaix, and took second at the most difficult race in the world, the super-mountainous Giro d'Italia. "Magnus is riding with climbers that weigh about a buck thirty," says Bourque. "He gives inspiration to anyone who once thought size matters."

HIGH-SPEED FOOD AND DRINK

The gear to keep fueled-up on the bike and run, for a song.

There is no bigger and more unnecessary momentum-wrecker than leaving the aero position to stop at a rural Circle K halfway through a long training day. It's unnecessary because slick tri-entrepreneurs have long produced a wide array of even slicker accessories that allow you to lug along enough extra food and drink for a family picnic without paying an aerodynamic price. Thanks to some legwork by my fellow *Triathlete Magazine* editor Jay Prasuhn, below are some of the clever creations that leave access to food and drink at your immediate disposal, and at $7 to $20, won't be a big burden on the bankroll.

Gel and drink flasks: Think of your grandpop's chrome whisky flask, only better. Not only do flasks allow quicker access to your gel (pulling open the cap instead of tearing off a top with your teeth and spitting it away) or drink, they're environmentally friendly. Just empty your gel packs into the flasks and throw the empty gel packet in the trash, not on the race course.

Flask belts: What better way to carry a water bottle worth of energy drink and a couple flasks of energy gel than around your waist (and out of your hands?). The even weight distribution keeps you focused on the run and off the sloshing and shifting of a water bottle in your hand.

Aero water bottles: Campagnolo used to make a sweet oval aero downtube bottle with a special cage. And now designers have bettered it for the triathlete with super-high-capacity beasts that slice through the wind like airfoils. Never before did drinking look so cool . . .

Here are some of the things available for each leg of a race, and where the designers have run wild:

On the Bike

In the drink category, **Profile Design** (www.profile-design.com) has a good grip. The AeroDrink System is a huge 32-ounce sharkfin-shaped bottle that sits in the open space of aftermarket aerobars. The open top allows you to pour in more bottles of your drink. You can now sip from the provided straw without having to reach for another bottle. Making a similar product is **Jetstream**, which features a little bit rounder bottle. For those who want to drink from a traditional bottle, but don't want it in the traditional main-triangle spot, Profile offers the Aqua Rack, a seatpost-mounted bracket that holds two bottles just under and behind the saddle, putting them in the aero slipstream behind the rider.

Since many race singlets don't have pockets, gel feeding on the bike is often difficult. To combat the problem, **DogHead Design** (www.dogheaddesign.com) came up with a clever gel flask holder (called the "Flask Whippet") that mounts to the bike top tube. The flask is Velcro-fastened to the bracket, and is at your immediate disposal in your cockpit. If Ironman Hawaii winners Lori Bowden and Luc Van Lierde both used this during the bike leg, there must be something to it.

In the case of food, we've seen the creative mold unwrapped pre-cut pieces of Power-bars to the top tube at Hawaii Ironman. Best done on a warm day when the bar is pliable. When that won't do the trick, **TNI USA** (www.tniusa.com) has three mesh aerobar bags capable of stashing bars, gels, and necessities like keys and money. The Air-box and Aeronet make space accomodation for that aero water bottle holder, while the Aero-pocket uses the entire void between the bars for storage.

On the Run

Fuelbelt (www.fuelbelt.com) holds eight five-ounce flasks with angled mouthpieces. The philosophy: carry the quantity of two large water bottles with the fluid distributed around the waist instead if shaking out of control while on the run. The mouthpiece is ideal for taking in either a gel or your favorite drink from the flask.

For those familiar with the more traditional gel-only flasks, The **Lava** (www.hy-trition.com) belt is a popular choice. Offered in different waist sizes, the wide elastic band secures with a tight Velcro seal, and the down-facing flasks are angled for an easy reach behind you, and since they're down-facing, you don't have to wait for the gel to drip to the mouthpiece; it's already there. An added pocket is available to stash your keys and cash.

For those who like taking standard gel packs along without the flask, TNI has the Energy Belt, an elastic belt with elastic slots capable of holding those packs. A mesh zipper packet at the back holds your keys and cash, and makes a great place to stash used packets (so don't throw them roadside, kids). A larger elastic loop can be used to pop vitamins, salt tablets, or other pills you might need in a film canister to take safely along with.

For those with an aversion to belts, DogHead Design makes several clip-on flask holders that clip easily to a strong waistband. But you like holding the flask by hand? DogHead Design chimes in again with the Flask Mitt, a small elastic strap that straps over your fingers with the flask in the palm of your hand, so you don't have to put a sweaty death grip on the flask for fear of dropping it.

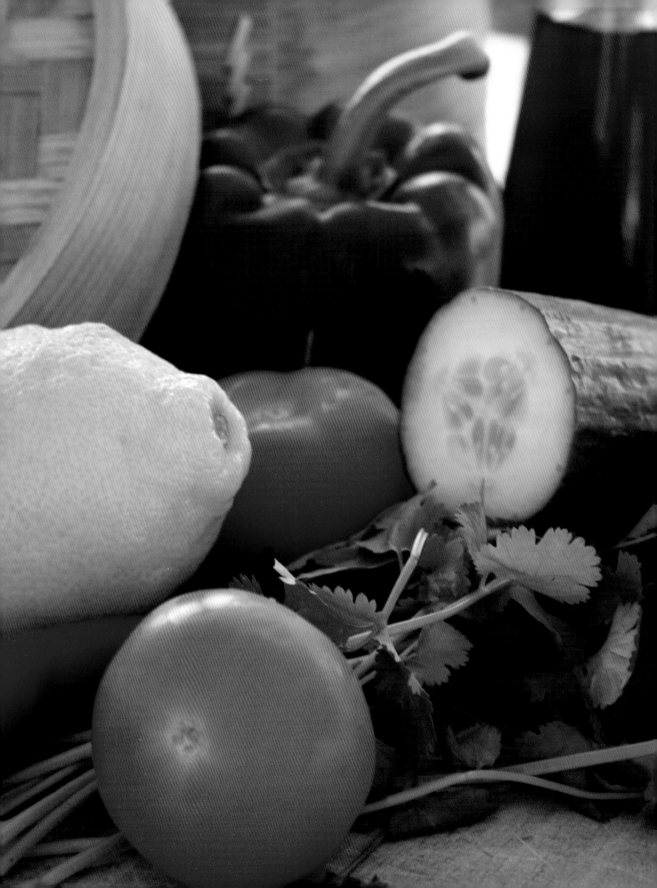

5
NUTRITIONAL OVERHAUL

HOW TO BANISH BAD FOODS, EAT FOR SPEED, LOVE SUPERFOODS, USE THE 30-MINUTE CARBOHYDRATE RECOVERY WINDOW, AND STAY HYDRATED

I recently spent some time talking with a man who is the brother of one of my coworkers. He's thirty-eight years old and is in a predicament similar to that of many Americans struggling with weight gain, the feelings associated with poor eating habits and a sedentary lifestyle, and the growing concern of being unhealthy and getting older, a potentially fatal pairing. A barber, his work hours are from noon to 8 PM. The bulk of his diet is composed of choices made at Burger King and a convenience store, the food all high in simple sugars, saturated fats, sodium, calories, and generally devoid of nutrition. We talked about triathlons and he said the idea of riding a motorcycle 12 miles sounds tiring to him, let alone the thought of being on a bicycle.

We talked at length, and I asked him specific questions about what he ate and when, and why he felt no energy. Right now he's in a pattern of sleeping until 11 in the morning. At work, he responds to hunger pangs by going to the convenience store to buy chips and "energy" drinks. At night, burgers and meat-laden pizza are his food choices. Soda is his drink of choice. He ends up being awake until three or four in the morning, falls asleep, and repeats the cycle all over.

I asked him how he felt. "I feel horrible all the time," he said. Considering his diet and disdain for physical activity, it wasn't a surprise.

He is trapped in a downward spiral that is easy to fall into. Cravings, malnutrition, and hopelessness are all words that accompany this spiral.

If you feel like you're trapped in this type of predicament, take heart in knowing you can be free of it. The prospect of training for and competing in a triathlon is a dynamic way to break out of the binding habits of an unhealthy lifestyle.

The Basic Training program, your first real entry into the triathlon world, begins in chapter 6. A critical part of this six-week introduction to the tri lifestyle will be your diet. We're making an assumption here that you need to/want to lose weight. If you fall into the description of the average American, then this will be the case. Again, a thorough discussion with

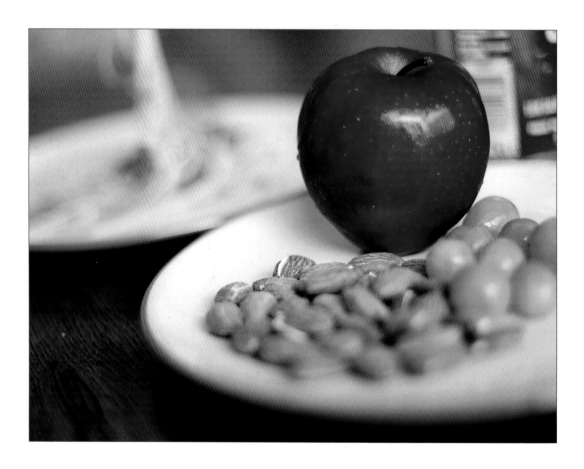

your doctor and a qualified dietician is the best way to assess where you're at in terms of health and what a smart target weight range is for you.

I. SETTING THE PHILOSOPHICAL TABLE

Before you rush out to the store for specific foods and start to plan new, healthier meals, you need to start with the right mindset. In other words, you must set the table before you bring out the food, figuratively and literally. Desire alone isn't enough to help you change long-ingrained eating habits. According to the American College of Sports Medicine, you must actively take steps to push your diet permanently in the right direction, overhaul your eating habits, and assume a healthier lifestyle. Rather than pursuing a quick fix, these recommendations are targeted at long-term alterations to your diet.

Cupboard cleanout. The ACSM suggests identifying the foods you overeat and keeping these foods to a bare minimum in your pantry.

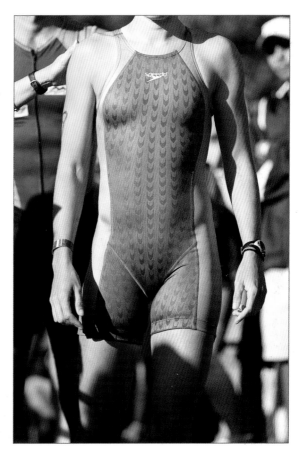

Don't restrict all foods all of the time. The ACSM says that evidence supports the idea that restricting items tends to lead us to overcompensate with other foods. It can be best to have the occasional treat rather than to eat too much of other things.

Listen to your body. Connect with your sense of hunger and when it strikes, and pay attention to when you do eat. Cultivate awareness. If you're prone to mindlessly chomping from a bowl of snacks, learn to tune into your true sense of hunger and how to satiate it with smart food choices, small portion sizes, and not skipping meals.

Learn portion sizes. More is not better. Don't bring home the message provided by TV commercials that you're getting a better deal for the dollar when your plate of food is mountainous. The ACSM suggests reading labels and gaining an understanding of what a serving size is.

Avoid drinking lots of calories. Again, get in the habit of reading labels. Even fruit juices can be heavy with calories. Fancy coffee drinks are now all the rage, but some of these contain whopping numbers of calories.

Frequency of eating out. The ACSM encourages limiting the number of times you eat out, no matter what kind of restaurant you frequent. This will help you establish more control over what you eat and how much.

And finally, maybe the most obvious one of all…

Stock up with healthy groceries. Common sense is a valuable commodity when it comes to engaging in a proper diet. You know that potato chips, fries, beer, triple-cheese pizza, and fudge are all examples of poor nutritional choices. Sometimes we end up eating that which we know is crap because it's abundant in American society. A powerful first step to countering this problem is to surround yourself with good foods. When you get hungry, instead of bolting to a fast-food joint, maybe you have a Lean Cuisine frozen dinner that you can microwave. Or maybe it's an apple and small bowl of low-fat cottage cheese. If the right food is nearby, you have the opportunity to break the bad habits that chain you to the fence post of being over-weight and feeling awful at the time.

II. SAFEWAY, HERE I COME

When you make your first pilgrimage to the grocery store as a budding triathlete, be sure to load up with the following types of food:

Produce: Fruits and vegetables should be consumed in abundance. The produce section has a vast array of selections available to you. Try and pick a variety of colors and foods for maximum nutritional impact.

Whole grains with minimal processing: Whole grain pastas, rice breads, and cereals will be the foundation of your fuel supply. When you have the choice, reach for the foods with the least amount of processing. (Examples: Whole grain bread versus white bread; regular oatmeal versus quick oats; brown rice instead of white rice). Look for high-fiber foods and avoid high-fat foods.

Canned foods: A plentiful stock of beans, vegetables, tomatoes, and fruit. Low-fat pasta sauces also go well on this shelf.

Meat, Fish, and Poultry: Lean cuts of meat, chicken, turkey, and fish are all in play. Avoid fried foods and select poulty without skin. Eating salmon once or twice a week will provide your body with omega-3 fatty acids, which have been shown to help reduce the risk of coronary heart disease.

Low-fat dairy foods: Low-fat or nonfat milk, yogurt, and reduced-calorie cheese are excellent choices, providing your body with calium, vitamin D, and protein. A cup of low-fat chocolate milk makes a nutritious desert.

Frozen dinners: Nutritionist Rebecca Marks Rudy says that the portion control and convenience of the right kind of frozen dinners (Healthy Choice, Lean Cuisine, Annie's, and the like) are a great thing to have in the freezer, especially if you lead a busy life. For example, let's say you end up working late and don't get home until past 7 PM. Rather than picking up a super-sized fast-food meal on the way home, you can opt to microwave a frozen dinner in five minutes or so.

III. BRING ON THE SUPERFOODS

Articles about so-called "superfoods" have been making a big splash at the newsstand these days, and for good reason: these foods are so jam-packed with nutrients and phytonutrients that you do yourself a disservice by not learning to love them. In case you've missed it, here are the stars of the trend and what they bring to the party:

- **Blueberries:** Antioxidants, antioxidants, and more antioxidants
- **Salmon:** Omega-3s
- **Broccoli:** Exploding with phytonutrients
- **Oats:** High in fiber
- **Oranges:** Antioxidants and phytonutrients
- **Watermelon:** Vitamin C and as much iron as spinach
- **Soy:** Pure nutritional magic
- **Spinach:** Of course—loaded with vitamins, iron, and more
- **Green tea:** Antioxidants, and a more subdued caffeine effect than coffee

Of course, the superfood universe is not limited to these garden-variety superstars. There are also romaine lettuce, green beans, whole-wheat spaghetti, and green, red, yellow, and orange bell peppers. And you may be surprised to discover that there are plenty of tasty, unconventional food products that are hidden right in front of your face, like sardines, mackerel, and prunes. They should rightfully bask in the glory of the superfood buzz, and can even serve as the centerpiece of a great prepared meal. Here are the unknown superfoods followed by a delicious recipe featuring each from *Cooking Light* magazine.

Sardines

Never thought you'd see the day when someone told you to eat sardines, did ya? Well, these little babies are a bountiful source of omega-3 fatty acids, a bulletproof vest when it comes to coronary heart disease and arthritis. Sardines also pack a healthy wallop of niacin and calcium.

Sardine Pâté Appetizers

    2 (3 3/4-ounce) cans sardines in water, drained
    1/4 cup finely chopped green onions
    1 1/2 prepared horseradish
    1 teaspoon dried dillweed
    1/4 cup plain nonfat yogurt
    1 tablespoon lemon juice
    30 pieces melba toast
    1/3 cup finely shredded carrot

Instructions: Place sardines in a bowl; mash with a fork. Add the next 5 ingredients, and stir well. Cover and chill for at least 2 hours. To serve, spoon 2 teaspoons pâté onto each melba toast; top with about 1/2 teaspoon carrot.

Yield: 2 1/2 dozen appetizers (serving size: 1 appetizer)

NUTRITION PER SERVING
CALORIES 30 (30% from fat); FAT 1g (sat 0.3g, mono 0.3g, poly 0.3g); PROTEIN 1.8g; CHOLESTEROL 4mg; CALCIUM 20mg; SODIUM 67mg; FIBER 0.1g; IRON 0.3mg; CARBOHYDRATE 3.4g

Mackerel

Like sardines, mackerel is another avenue toward the healthful land of omega-3 fatty acid intake. (Studies first conducted in the 1970s linked the positive benefits of a diet rich in omega-3s to the Inuits of Greenland, a native culture subsisting on seal and whale meat.) Mackerel is also rich in selenium, an antioxidant (antioxidants are big names in the superfood aisle).

Mackerel Pâté Appetizers

Same recipe as above; simply replace mackerel for sardines.

Walnuts

Almonds have been getting the superfood headlines, but let's not forget their crunchy little brother. Studies have shown that the polyphenolic compounds ellagic and gallic acid, found in walnuts, are bad news for free radical damage. Additionally, a 2003 study published in the journal *Phytochemistry* gave kudos to the walnut as being so rich with antioxidant activity they called the powerful little snack "remarkable." A handful of walnuts and almonds a day keeps the heart surgeon away.

Pear, Walnut, and Blue Cheese Salad with Cranberry Vinaigrette

Cranberry sauce, the base for the vinaigrette, lends a holiday flavor to this salad. You can make and refrigerate the dressing up to a week ahead.

Vinaigrette
   1/2 cup canned whole-berry cranberry sauce
   1/4 cup fresh orange juice (about 1 orange)
   1 tablespoon olive oil
   2 tablespoons balsamic vinegar
   1 teaspoon sugar
   1 teaspoon minced peeled fresh ginger
   1/4 teaspoon salt

Salad
   18 Bibb lettuce leaves (about 2 heads)
   2 cups sliced peeled pear (about 2 pears)
   2 tablespoons fresh orange juice
   1 cup (1/8-inch-thick) slices red onion, separated into rings
   1/3 cup (2 ounces) crumbled blue cheese
   2 tablespoons coarsely chopped walnuts, toasted

To prepare the vinaigrette, place the first 7 ingredients in a medium bowl; stir well with a whisk.

To prepare the salad, divide the lettuce leaves evenly among 6 salad plates. Toss pear with 2 tablespoons orange juice. Divide pear and onion evenly among leaves. Top each serving with about 1 tablespoon cheese and 1 teaspoon walnuts. Drizzle each serving with about 2 1/2 tablespoons vinaigrette.

Yield: 6 servings

NUTRITION PER SERVING
CALORIES 148 (38% from fat); FAT 6.3g (sat 1.8g, mono 2.5g, poly 1.5g); PROTEIN 2.7g; CHOLESTEROL 5mg; CALCIUM 60mg; SODIUM 205mg; FIBER 2.4g; IRON 0.4mg; CARBOHYDRATE 22.3g

Tofu

Tofu is the odd looking white gelatinous material and maybe the last thing a sane person might imagine to be the product of beans (soybeans, to be specific). When well-tended, protein-thick tofu can be tasty, and its culinary uses are many. Tofu can also reduce the risk of heart disease by lowering LDL cholesterol.

Broccoli-Tofu Stir-Fry

This simple meatless stir-fry has a subtle yet addictive sauce. To cut preparation time, use precut broccoli florets. They're near the salad greens in the supermarkets.

1 (3 1/2-ounce) bag boil-in-bag brown rice
2 tablespoons low-sodium soy sauce
2 tablespoons oyster sauce
2 1/2 teaspoons cornstarch
2 teaspoons rice vinegar
2 teaspoons dark sesame oil
2 teaspoons vegetable oil
1 pound firm tofu, drained and cut into 1/2-inch cubes
1/4 teaspoon salt
2 cups broccoli florets
3/4 cup water
1 1/2 tablespoons bottled minced garlic

Cook the rice according to package directions.

While rice cooks, combine soy sauce and the next 4 ingredients (soy sauce through sesame oil) in a small bowl, stirring with a whisk; set aside.

Heat vegetable oil in a large nonstick skillet over medium-high heat. Add the tofu, and sprinkle with salt. Cook 8 minutes or until golden brown, tossing frequently. Remove tofu from pan, and keep warm. Add broccoli, water, and garlic to pan. Cover and cook 4 minutes or until crisp-tender, stirring occasionally. Uncover; add soy sauce mixture and tofu, stirring gently to coat. Cook 2 minutes or until sauce thickens, stirring occasionally. Serve the broccoli mixture over rice.

Yield: 4 servings (serving size: 1 cup stir-fry and 1/2 cup rice)

NUTRITION PER SERVING
CALORIES 451 (17% from fat); FAT 8.3g (sat 1.4g, mono 2.6g, poly 3.8g); PROTEIN 16.2g; CHOLESTEROL 0.0mg; CALCIUM 87mg; SODIUM 581mg; FIBER 4.4g; IRON 2.8mg; CARBOHYDRATE 78g

Prunes

They're not just for Grandpa. Regardless of your age, prunes are a terrific source of iron and fiber. Ounce for ounce prunes are higher in fiber than beans, and are a good source of beta-carotene and potassium. Maybe not the fruit you want to have waiting for you in your special needs bag, but suitable for most other occasions.

Prune Wake-up Shake
    3/4 cup prune juice, chilled
    3/4 cup 2% reduced-fat milk, chilled
    1/2 cup vanilla low-fat yogurt

3/4 teaspoon vanilla extract
Dash of ground allspice
8 bite-size pitted prunes
1 ripe banana, cut into chunks

Combine all ingredients in a blender; process until smooth. Serve immediately.

Yield: 3 servings (serving size: 1 cup)

NUTRITION PER SERVING
CALORIES 215 (11% from fat); FAT 2.6g (sat 1.1g, mono 1.1g, poly 0.3g); PROTEIN 4.9g; CHOLESTEROL 7mg; CALCIUM 161mg; SODIUM 71mg; FIBER 1.9g; IRON 1.5mg; CARBOHYDRATE 45.2g

Garlic

With a strong reputation for being good for the blood, garlic has also been linked with helping to prevent cancer, heart disease, and arthritis. On a lighter note, it rejuvenates your skin. Not to be forgotten, a little dexterity with the garlic crusher can give your overall diet a tasty zap.

Baked Lemon–Garlic Chicken with Bell Peppers

Sauce
    3/4 cup fresh lemon juice (about 6 lemons)
    3/4 cup fat-free Italian dressing
    1/2 teaspoon freshly ground black pepper
    3 garlic cloves, minced

Chicken
    2 cups (1/4-inch) red bell pepper strips
    1 cup (1/4-inch) green bell pepper strips
    1 cup (1/4-inch) yellow bell pepper strips
    3 chicken breast halves (about 1 1/2 pounds)
    3 chicken leg quarters (about 1 1/2 pounds)
    12 (1/8-inch-thick) slices lemon (about 1 lemon)
    Cooking spray

To prepare the sauce, combine the first 4 ingredients in a medium bowl, stirring with a whisk. Cover and chill 1/2 cup sauce.

To prepare the chicken, combine remaining 1 cup sauce, bell peppers, and chicken in a large bowl, and toss to coat. Cover chicken mixture, and refrigerate for 4 hours or overnight.

Preheat oven to 400 degrees.

Remove chicken from bowl, and discard the sauce. Loosen the skin from the breast halves and leg quarters by inserting fingers, gently pushing between the skin and meat. Insert 2 lemon slices under loosened skin of each chicken piece. Place the chicken pieces, loosened skin sides up, on a broiler pan coated with cooking spray. Spread the bell peppers on broiler pan around chicken. Bake at 400 degrees for 50 minutes or until the chicken is done. Remove the skin from the chicken. Arrange chicken and bell peppers on a platter, and keep warm.

Place 1/2 cup chilled sauce in a small saucepan, and cook over medium heat 3 minutes or until warm. Pour warm sauce over the baked chicken and bell peppers.

Yield: 6 servings (serving size: 1 chicken piece, 1/3 cup bell peppers, and about 1 tablespoon sauce)

NUTRITION PER SERVING
CALORIES 216 (28% from fat); FAT 6.7g (sat 1.8g, mono 2.4g, poly 1.6g); PROTEIN 30.2g; CHOLESTEROL 91mg; CALCIUM 28mg; SODIUM 385mg; FIBER 1.7g; IRON 1.7mg; CARBOHYDRATE 9g

Barley

Another fiber-rich food, whole-grain barley fills you up with iron and powerful cancer-preventative phytochemicals. Good as your bowl of cereal in the morning, barley is also a smart substitute for pasta.

Barley "Pasta" Salad

The flavor and texture of barley is similar to that of pasta, so we combined it with the typical pasta salad ingredients.

    2 cups water
    1/2 cup uncooked pearl barley
    2 tablespoons fresh lemon juice
    1 tablespoon olive oil
    1/2 teaspoon salt
    2 cups finely chopped seeded tomato
    1 cup thinly sliced spinach
    1/2 cup finely chopped green bell pepper
    1/2 cup chopped seeded peeled cucumber
    1/2 cup (2 ounces) diced part-skim mozzarella cheese
    1/4 cup finely chopped pepperoncini peppers
    2 teaspoons dry oregano

Bring 2 cups water to a boil in a large saucepan. Add barley; cover, reduce heat, and simmer 45 minutes. Drain and rinse with cold water; drain.

Combine the juice, oil, and salt in large bowl; stir well with a whisk. Add barley, tomato, and remaining ingredients; toss gently to coat.

Yield: **5 servings** (serving size: about 1 cup)

NUTRITION PER SERVING
CALORIES 153 (31% from fat); FAT 5.2g (sat 1.6g, mono 2.6g, poly 0.6g); PROTEIN 6g; CHOLESTEROL 7mg; CALCIUM 107mg; SODIUM 436mg; FIBER 5g; IRON 1.8mg; CARBOHYDRATE 22.4g

Yams

Pass by the russet potatoes next time you're in the fruit and vegetable aisle, and pick up some flavorful yams instead. Studies indicate that the wealthy amount of carotenes in yams will bolster your defense against the growth of tumors, as well as help protect you against heart disease.

Sweet Potato–Pecan Pancakes

You can use 3/4 cup mashed winter squash instead of the sweet potatoes, if desired.

    1 1/4 cups all-purpose flour
    1/4 cup chopped pecans, toasted and divided
    2 1/4 teaspoons baking powder
    1 teaspoon pumpkin-pie spice
    1/4 teaspoon salt
    1 cup fat-free milk
    1/4 cup packed dark brown sugar
    1 tablespoon vegetable oil
    1 teaspoon vanilla extract
    2 large eggs, lightly beaten
    1 (16-ounce) can sweet potatoes or yams, drained and mashed (about 3/4 cup)

Lightly spoon flour into dry measuring cups; level with a knife. Combine flour, 2 tablespoons pecans, baking powder, pumpkin-pie spice, and salt in a large bowl. Combine milk and next 4 ingredients (milk through eggs); add to flour mixture, stirring until smooth. Stir in sweet potatoes.

Spoon about 1/4 cup batter onto a hot nonstick griddle or large nonstick skillet. Turn pancakes when tops are covered with bubbles and edges look cooked. Sprinkle pancakes with 2 tablespoons pecans.

Yield: **6 servings** (serving size: 2 pancakes and 1 teaspoon pecans)

Kidney Beans

Mix kidney beans (and most any other beans, to be frank) with rice, and you have yourself a practically fat-free protein, vegetarian through and through. Kidney beans are loaded with fiber, and will lower the glycemic rating of any meal you make them a part of. Kidney beans are high in folate, manganese, iron, and vitamin B1.

All-American Chili

> 6 ounces hot turkey Italian sausage
> 2 cups chopped onion
> 1 cup chopped green bell pepper
> 8 garlic cloves, minced
> 1 pound ground sirloin
> 1 jalapeño pepper, chopped
> 2 tablespoons chili powder
> 2 tablespoons brown sugar
> 1 tablespoon ground cumin
> 3 tablespoons tomato paste
> 1 teaspoon dried oregano
> 1/2 teaspoon freshly ground black pepper
> 1/4 teaspoon salt
> 2 bay leaves
> 1 1/4 cups Merlot or other fruity red wine
> 2 (28-ounce) cans whole tomatoes, undrained and coarsely chopped
> 2 (15-ounce) cans kidney beans, drained
> 1/2 cup (2 ounces) shredded reduced-fat sharp cheddar cheese

Heat a large Dutch oven over medium-high heat. Remove casings from sausage. Add sausage, onion, and the next 4 ingredients (onion through jalapeño) to pan; cook 8 minutes or until sausage and beef are browned, stirring to crumble.

Add chili powder and the next 7 ingredients (chili powder through bay leaves), and cook for 1 minute, stirring constantly. Stir in wine, tomatoes, and kidney beans; bring to a boil. Cover, reduce heat, and simmer 1 hour, stirring occasionally.

Uncover and cook for 30 minutes, stirring occasionally. Discard the bay leaves. Sprinkle each serving with cheddar cheese.

Note: Like most chilis, this version tastes even better the next day.

Yield: 8 servings (serving size: 1 1/4 cups chili and 1 tablespoon cheese)

NUTRITION PER SERVING
CALORIES 375 (29% from fat); FAT 12g (sat 4.6g, mono 4.1g, poly 1.1g); PROTEIN 28.9g; CHOLESTEROL 59mg; CALCIUM 165mg; SODIUM 969mg; FIBER 8.2g; IRON 5mg; CARBOHYDRATE 33.7g

IV. FIVE TIPS TO TAILOR YOUR DIET TO YOUR TRAINING

Now that you've discovered what kinds of foods to buy and ingest on a daily basis, you need to know how and when and how many of them to eat. Specifically, you need an eating strategy that will keep you properly fueled for the unique demands of triathlon training. Keep in mind that a training session not only jacks up your calorie burning, requiring you to eat more than a sedentary person on a diet, but also requires specific types of calories at a certain time to prepare for and maximize a quality training session and a quality recovery.

The following fueling tips come courtesy of sports nutritionist and exercise physiologist Kim S. Brown, MS, RD, a frequent and valued contributor to *Triathlete Magazine*.

Tip #1: Don't short your daily calorie intake. Otherwise, you won't have enough fuel in the tank to avoid muscle breakdown.

It's easy to underestimate your energy demands during training, especially if you are beginner triathlete trying to lose weight—but beware of eating too little. Inadequate fuel in your tank degrades the full benefits from your training and can actually heighten your risk for injury.

Depending on daily training volume and intensity, most triathletes require a range of 16 to 30 calories per pound of lean body weight; male triathletes training for long-course triathlons require the latter end of these requirements. Here's how that translates into real numbers: As a 110-pound female with approximately 15 percent body fat, I generally consume about 2,500 calories a day during Ironman training. I split my 2,500-calorie daily intake into four to six 400- to 600-calorie meals, consisting of combinations of carbohydrate and protein and a lot of colorful fruits and vegetables.

Important: Keep in mind that my 2,500 calories per day is my baseline of regular meals only and DOES NOT include calories that I consume while working out and immediately after working out. That will be discussed later.

Whether your calorie baseline is 2,500 or 4,000, its breakdown between carbs, protein, and fat should not change. You should aim at a balance of 55 to 60 percent healthy carbohydrates (fruits, vegetables, whole grains, beans), 15 to 20 percent lean protein (soy, low-fat dairy, chicken breast, fish, round steak, turkey) and 20 to 25 percent healthy fats (avocado, nuts, seeds, olives). Remember to spread out your total calorie needs into four to six smaller meals throughout the day. Do not avoid or restrict major food groups (e.g., carbohydrate-restricted diets); unbalanced meal patterns can hurt performance and have potentially serious health consequences.

For those interested in losing weight, a few special rules apply: Never restrict your diet by more than 1,000 calories per day; this causes an energy drain and muscle breakdown. A restriction of 250 to 500 calories each day from your norm will help you lose a half pound to one pound of fat mass a week. On the flipside, if you need to gain body weight, boost your calorie intake by 250 calories daily.

A typical day of eating for me includes:

Breakfast: Oatmeal blended with granola, berries, almonds, and milk along with Naked Juice.

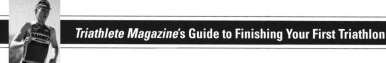
Lunch: Vegetarian turkey sandwich with lettuce, tomato, and cheese on whole grain bread, vegetable soup or salad, a piece of fruit, and low-fat chocolate milk.

Afternoon snack: Fruit smoothie prepared with yogurt, juice, and frozen fruit, or an energy bar and piece of fruit.

Dinner: Large salad plus a pasta dish prepared with soy meat.

Evening Snack: Small bowl of granola with almonds and nonfat milk.

Tip #2: Stay hydrated all the time.

Drink half your body weight (pounds) in fluid ounces each day. That's not as easy as it sounds. If you weigh 180 pounds, that means you ought to drink 90 fluid ounces a day—nearly three quarts. It does not include your morning cup of joe or any other caffeinated beverage, but it does include any fluid such as juice, milk, and broth.

Pre-workout hydration: In the hour or two before your ride, run, or swim, top off the tank with a full water bottle (approximately 16–24 oz).

During the workout: Aim for 5 to 12 ounces of fluid every 20 minutes. Carry a water bottle or fuel belt if necessary. On workouts over 90 minutes, use an electrolyte sports drink.

Post-workout: Rehydrate with a sports drink if you find your urine color tending toward a bright-yellow color rather than clear, or if you have lost a significant amount of weight (one pound or more).

Tip #3: Pre-load big, hard workouts.

Don't embark on a strenuous workout—either high-intensity or long-duration (more than 90 minutes) or both—without a full tank of gas. Otherwise, you might run out before you're done.

Remember these numbers: Consume half your lean body weight in carbohydrate grams for every hour before your workout starts. For most female triathletes, this equates to 45 to 60 grams of carbohydrates (approximately 200–250 calories) in the hour before. A sample snack: An energy bar, or a piece of whole grain toast spread lightly with peanut butter with one sliced banana.

For most male triathletes, it equates to 60 to 75 grams of carbohydrate (approximately 250–300 calories) an hour before your workout. Example snack: A banana and an energy bar, or a small bowl of Special K cereal topped with strawberries and nonfat milk with a glass of orange juice.

General rules: Minimize the amount of fiber, protein, and fat in the meal, since these three nutrients will slow down digestion and potentially cause gastrointestinal problems (e.g., diarrhea) during your workout. Also, drink fluids with your meal to ensure optimal absorption of the nutrients.

Tip #4: Refuel when training goes over 90 minutes.

Keep in mind that your body has unlimited stores of fat, but limited stores of carbohydrates, which are essential to athletic performance and a whole range of key bodily functions.

Therefore, your goal on long training sessions—over 90 minutes (which are frequent during training for Ironman and half Ironman races)—is to try to "optimize" fuel use; that is, burn your fat and save your carbs. To do the latter, you must refuel with carbs on long workouts. Every hour past 90 minutes, ingest a 1/2-gram of carbs plus an 1/8-gram of protein per pound of lean body weight. This keeps your carbs from bottoming out, and helps rebuild your battered muscles, which are made of protein. Opt for sports food containing small amounts of protein (Accelerade, Perpetuem, energy bars) when training for long-course triathlons.

The numbers: For most females, the formula works out to ingesting 45 to 60 grams of carbohydrate after 90 minutes. That might be one energy gel chased with electrolyte-enhanced water every half hour.

Male triathletes require an hourly dose of 60 to 75 grams of carbohydrates after 90 minutes. Sample: One energy gel with electrolyte-enhanced water, plus eight ounces of a sports drink every half hour.

Tip #5: The 30-minute window: for best recovery after hard training efforts, get your carbo-protein combo down fast.

Get used to the term "the 30-minute window." It means that the body is uniquely open to restocking its depleted stores within a half hour of finishing exercise. In other words, by the next day, your recovery will be much more complete if you ate before the window closed.

Your goal: try to consume a 1/2-gram of carbohydrate and an 1/8-gram of protein per pound of lean body weight.

How that translates: female triathletes should down a 200- to 250-calorie snack, and males 300-plus calories.

What to eat: sports food, real food, or both. Post-workout recovery foods might include low-fat chocolate milk, smoothies with a protein boost, peanut butter/honey/banana sandwiches, salted pretzels dipped in yogurt, and cottage cheese/fruit combinations. Meal replacement shakes like Boost and Ensure provide a convenient nutritional punch too.

V. MORE ON THE 30-MINUTE WINDOW: WHY RELOADING IS KEY TO RAPID RECOVERY

To optimize performance, an endurance athlete must keep his body strong, his energy high, and his immune system healthy. Technically, the 30-minute window following hard effort is crucial because it is when the body's sensitivity to insulin is at its highest, and when muscles are able to quickly absorb nutrients for maximum restoration and storage of muscle glycogen. Of course, getting proper nutrition and hydration is essential before, during, and after you cross the finish line, but the "after" is crucial. Below, Mary Ellen Bingham, MS, RD, CDN, a nutrition associate for Trismarter.com, explains why reloading is so essential to recovery.

With training periods of triathletes typically less than 24 hours apart, you must consume food with 30 minutes that maximizes your rehydration and nutritional recovery to replace muscle fuel for the next workout. Specifically, you aim to replenish muscle glycogen, body water (hydration), and electrolytes (primarily sodium).

What to ingest? Carbs, immediately. After all, an athlete's body can be depleted of muscle glycogen rather quickly. Studies suggest 0.5–0.7 grams per pound of body weight (1–1.2 g/kg) is an optimal goal for rapidly absorbed carbohydrate intake. So, a 155-pound athlete (70 kg) may require about 80 grams of carb after a long training session.

A common, but debated, practice is a 3:1 or 4:1 ratio of carbohydrate to protein for your recovery nutrition. Choose high-quality protein sources: whey protein, dairy products and soy milk, lean meats, or nuts to speed up the repair of muscle tissue. If the 155-pound athlete is consuming 80 grams of carbohydrate, get at least 20 grams of protein. Additionally, glutamine, an amino acid, is found in many recovery products and may be beneficial for muscle repair.

Water weight: Replace each pound during the workout lost with 24 ounces of fluid. Add sodium to enhance rehydration and replace sweat-loss. Options: Salty snacks, salt packets, and sports drinks. The recommendation is 110–200 milligrams of sodium per 8 ounces of fluid. The sodium content of various sports drinks per 8 ounces is as follows: Gatorade—110 mg, Accelerade—115 mg, Gatorade Endurance—200 mg.

Solid or liquid replacement? As long as you stay within 30 minutes, it's all up to you. What you take often depends on taste, tolerance, convenience, and affordability. Some athletes can't tolerate solid food immediately following exercise. Try recovery mixes—a bit expensive, but good at a 3:1 or 4:1 ratio, and adequate fluid and sodium to match your losses. Examples: Recoverite by Hammer Nutrition—332 calories, 65 g carbohydrate, 20 g protein, 148 mg sodium, and 38 mg potassium in 4 scoops, mixed with 16–24 ounces of water. Sports drinks, commonly used for recovery, are good, cheap sources of sodium and fluid replacement. New Gatorade Endurance offers 90 more mg sodium per 8 ounces, and Accelerade offers 4 grams of protein per 8 ounces.

Choices for recovery foods seem endless. Lots of options: sports drinks and recovery mixes, energy bars, whole foods, fruit juices, and the latest superfood fad, low-fat (1%) chocolate milk. The latter is very successful, with 84 grams of carbohydrate, 26 grams of protein, 2 grams of fat, and 345 mg of sodium in 24 ounces! This meets your recovery needs a bit better than a Big Mac (540 calories, 25 g protein, 75 mg cholesterol, 30 g fat [10 g saturated fat], 1,040 mg sodium, and 45 g carbs)! Other great real food choices include a turkey sandwich with pretzels, a bagel with peanut butter and jelly, a fruit/granola/yogurt parfait, or even a smoothie made with fresh or frozen fruit, soy or low fat milk, and yogurt. Just be sure to wash these foods down with and appropriate amount of water.

Now, meet the two-hour window: Even after filling the 30-minute window, your body is still recovering for two hours after the session. Eat a balanced meal, packed with protein, vegetables, and a large portion of starch. Try to get some "healthy" fats (mono- and poly-unsaturated). Example of healthy and balanced meals include salmon with sweet potato and steamed vegetables or pasta with chicken and vegetables mixed with olive oil and a little garlic salt and parmesan cheese for flavor.

VI. WATER WORLD: BASIC RULES OF PROPER HYDRATION

How much do I drink? What do I drink? These are key questions for any triathlete—beginner and veteran alike. After all, appropriate fluid intake before, during, and after exercise is an important predictor of athletic performance. Dehydration can wreck your day. Hyper-hydration—too much water and too little electrolytes—can threaten your life. You'll understand why quickly if you know some fast facts:

- Water is essential to the human body
- 60–70 percent of our body mass is water
- Up to 90 percent of our brain mass is water
- Up to 75 percent of muscle is comprised of water
- Water is the main component of blood—the important carrier of glucose, oxygen and other nutrients

As you can see, water is everywhere in the human body. Take a lot of it away, and something will change and get out of balance—and not for the better.

So, back to the original question: How much should I drink?

In general, before training even starts, your body loses 64-80 ounces of water daily through urine, feces, sweat, skin, and expired air. You must replace this amount—between two and three quarts of fluid—every day.

Surprising, isn't it? You must hydrate even if all you do is sit around all day. So what about exercise? How do hydration requirements rise when you factor in often-rigorous training?

Of course, a scientific formula based on body weight has been designed to calculate individual needs. For moderately active men and women, multiply body weight in pounds by 0.35 or 0.31, respectively, to calculate fluid requirements in ounces per day. For example, for a 175-pound man: $175 \times 0.35 = 61.25$ ounces (a little over 7 cups of fluid daily); or for a 125-pound woman: $125 \times 0.31 = 38.75$ ounces (almost 5 cups of fluid daily).

Another, albeit much less scientific, way to determine daily fluid requirements is to evaluate your urine. Dark and concentrated urine is indicative of inadequate fluid intake. Urine should be pale yellow to clear, and copious.

Just as you would "carbo-load" before embarking on a long training ride or run, you should also "aqua-load."

The American College of Sports Medicine and National Athletic Trainers Association recommends that athletes should be well hydrated before beginning endurance exercise. The day before a long training session or race, aim to drink as much as ninety ounces of fluid along with a diet high in carbohydrates with at least three grams of sodium. Two to three hours before the event, drink 400 to 600 mililiters (13 to 20 ounces) and during the event aim to drink 150 to 350 mililiters (5 to 12 ounces) every 15 to 20 minutes (totaling 400–800 mL or 12–24 ounces per hour).

But beware of overdrinking. Consuming more than 800 milliliters per hour will increase your risk for hyponatremia. Hyponatremia is the opposite of dehydration. It is a serious electrolyte disturbance resulting from water intoxication.

These recommendations are general and suggest a very wide range for adequate fluid consumption. A good way to calculate your personal fluid requirements during exercise is to calculate sweat losses by weighing yourself unclothed, then exercising (put your clothes back on!) without consuming any fluids or food for one hour, and then reweigh after exercise without your sweaty clothes on. For every pound (16 ounces) lost, you need to drink 80 to 100 percent—for example, if you lose one pound in one hour you should aim to drink 13 to 16 ounces of fluid per hour (390–480 mL).

What should you drink? Three basic rules apply:

- Water is the best beverage choice for sub one-hour training sessions and races.
- For events over one hour, drink electrolyte beverages with 4 to 8 percent carbohydrates.
- Don't drink coffee or caffeine-containing drinks; they may interfere with sleep patterns and will have a mild diuretic effect.

Don't forget to drink when your training session or race is over. Post-exercise fluid intake is critical for proper recovery. Aim to consume up to 150 percent of weight lost during an exercise session, or 24 ounces per pound lost. Generally, athletes will lose 1 to 2 percent of their body weight—loss exceeding 2 percent is an indicator of dehydration. To calculate fluid replacement without weighing yourself, use the following example: A 135-pound woman will lose approximately 1.35 pounds (21.6 ounces) during exercise; she should aim to replace 100 to 150 percent of 21.6 (or 24 ounces per 1.35 pounds = 21 to 32 ounces of fluid) during recovery. The best recovery beverage is a combination of water, carbohydrates, and electrolytes, such as sports drinks or juice, to replace both lost fluid and glycogen.

Bottom line: Adequate fluid intake before, during, and after exercise will aid in peak athletic performance and recovery. In the heat of triathlon training in spring and summer, and with temperatures generally increasing with global warming, it is vital to consume adequate fluids to prevent dehydration. In chapter 12, Race Day, we get into the specifics of what to eat and drink during competition. In the mean time, let the information here be your guide to safe and productive fueling during your regular training schedule.

6

BASIC TRAINING

THE SIX-WEEK ON-RAMP TO THE ATHLETE HIGHWAY

When you're just starting out, it can be intimidating to be in the presence of an exceptionally fit triathlete. Don't be. The truth is, many triathletes have at one point been fat and out of shape. Ask them their story, and you'll likely hear the most satisfying part about being a triathlete was in the their first months of training. It's the best part. The transformation from nonathlete to athlete, or regaining an athleticism lost after high school, is about gaining back control of your life. It's about setting yourself free from a prison built of bad habits, like too much junk food consumed in front of too much television, and enjoying the drama of improving yourself, feeling the improvement on a day-to-day basis, and in the end accomplishing something as remarkable as being able to identify yourself as a competitive triathlete.

If you wish your physical transformation could happen overnight, extinguish that thought. The best part about your journey is going to be the first few months, using each day to get a little bit better, and through the miracle of consistency and virtue of patience, realizing goals you never thought were possible. If you could take a pill and make something like this happen overnight, you would miss the point. The deepest satisfaction you'll ever receive from triathlon will come from the knowledge that you slowly, steadily performed an act of self-discipline and dedication, and that the rewards of crossing the finish line and earning a finisher's medal were just the icing on the cake.

Here's one of the best parts about committing yourself to endurance athletics: the satisfaction you will gain will not come from the subjective arena. We live in a world where sales and marketing dominate the culture, where subjective opinion often has more power than objective fact. When we are praised for some quality or talent, it's hard to feel good about it if the praise is staked in subjective thought or if the person whipping out the compliments is just being nice, not necessarily truthful. When you perform a workout and jot it down into your logbook, it's a real accomplishment. When you complete your first three weeks of training, it's a real accomplishment. When you eventually cross the finish line of your first triathlon, you will know exactly what you did and you can be proud of it. In other words, there's no bullshit involved.

The following six-week program is designed for the person who needs to start off at the very beginning. You need to strengthen your bones, muscles, and connective tissue and toughen your mind for the more rigorous training that will follow. So your initial six weeks will begin with walking and work toward walk-jogging. You will also perform your first bike and swim workouts. The heart of this program is the implementation of several basic nutrition habits that will begin to restore your health, provide you with more energy, and help you lose unnecessary weight.

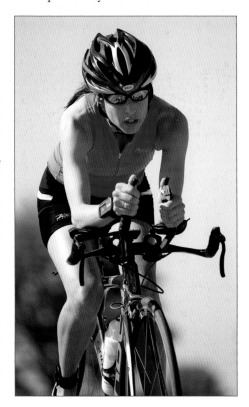

This program is general in nature, and if the consultation with your doctor reveals you have serious weight and health issues, you will need to work with your doctor to modify this program so that it will be safe and effective. Only with your doctor's okay is it safe to begin the following program. If you have a serious obesity issue, or if you have worries about your health and what specifically to do about it, consulting with the doctors and coaches at Trismarter.com will help you identify specific needs and map out a safe, specific plan.

THE CORE PRINCIPLES

Briefly, before we jump into the six-week training program, be aware of the core training principles that will help you progress through it swiftly and injury-free. We will touch on the following basic concepts many times throughout your program.

1. **The principle of gradual progression**

   If you think that fitness is gained by ambushing the local gym and training until you collapse on a treadmill, forget this image. When you are introducing your body to exercise and also to a training program, it's best to start easy and slowly work up. Even when you're super fit, the bulk of training should be aerobic. The most effective work you can do in the early stages of a training program is low-key aerobic conditioning, coaxing your heart rate into a range of approximately 60 percent of what might be your maximum effort. If you're running or biking, being in an aerobic training zone means you should be able to pass the "talk test"—you should be able to comfortably carry on a conversation with a training partner. Spending time consistently in this zone on a weekly basis will, over time and in tune with the principle of gradual progression, yield powerful effects.

2. **The principle of recovery**

   Recovery and restoration of your body after an exercise session is when your improvement takes place. You stress the system and then rest the system, and during the rest

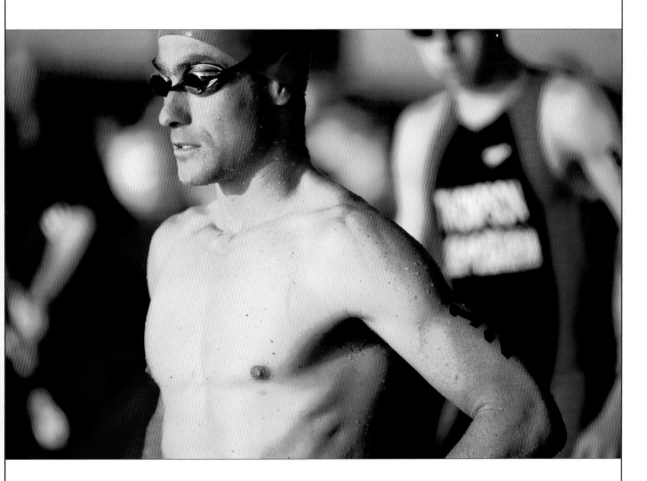

phase the body will naturally adapt to the new stresses being placed upon it—meaning you get stronger. So if you have three training days a week, it's best to spread them out to make use of proper recovery cycles. For example, training Monday, Wednesday, and Saturday.

3. **The principle of specificity**

   The principle of specificity states that to improve in an activity, you must practice that activity in the way it is ultimately to be performed. To become a better runner, for example, you must run. To swim the freestyle better, you must spend some time swimming freestyle. To perform a long-distance race, you must incorporate some long-distance training.

4. **The principle of variety**

   Yes, you must do the specific work required by the event you're training for, but it would be a mistake to wake up and race a triathlon everyday. It's good to mix up workouts, perform training in different places, and keep free of ruts where you do repeat the same old workouts month after month.

5. **The principle of focused attention**

   Want to make rapid progress as an athlete? Then give each and every workout a goal, one that you are accountable for through the medium of a detailed logbook. The key to building true momentum in your training plan is this: Put in the work and record everything you can about it. Use tools of measurement to mark this progress (body fat measurement,

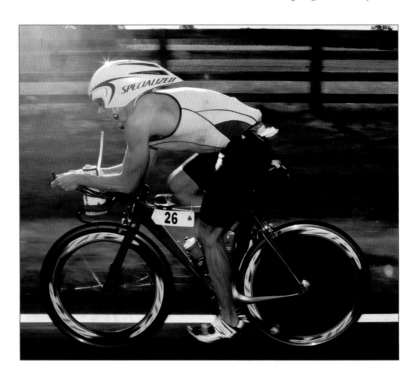

weight, photographs of yourself, etc.). This measurement will verify the increments of improvement. As you witness this payoff, the motivation to train doubles.

6. **Lose weight through diet and keep it off with training**

    This is in fact the strategy employed by the expert coaches and dieticians at Trismarter .com, a triathlon coaching company. For clients having to overcome a weight problem starting out, Trismarter.com focuses on diet for the first stage of the program to initiate weight loss, and then adds the additional angle of endurance exercise to keep it off. You too will begin by making a few simple adjustments to your diet as you carefully ease into a triathlon-training program. Unlike dieting alone, the one-two punch of diet and exercise *does* help you keep weight off as you establish an enjoyable lifestyle as a triathlete.

7. **The principle of simplicity**

    The principle of simplicity should be employed if you are brand-new to any discipline. Avoid overreaching with your goals. Keep things calm and basic, and proceed in small, well-defined steps. When things get too complicated, it becomes easy to quit in frustration. Rather, start slow and be patient. Over the course of time, through incremental steps, you will pick up all the necessary details to become a complete triathlete.

    With simplicity in mind, get your doctor's okay to workout, and get ready for good food and good movement. It's time for the Basic Training program.

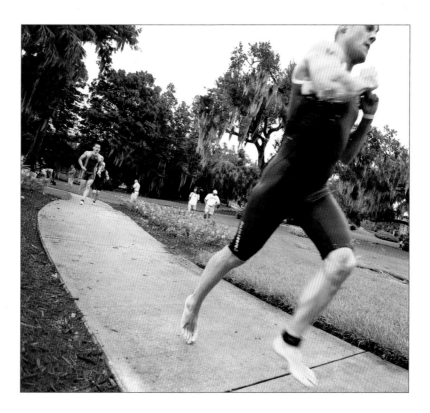

THE SIX-WEEK BASIC TRAINING PROGRAM

Week 1

Objectives:

1. Each day, take a fast-paced walk for 10 minutes or more, breaking a sweat and notice-ably increasing respiration.
2. Eat a "power" breakfast each day.
3. Record your results for objectives 1 and 2 in a notebook.

By the way, what's a "power" breakfast? Simply, a can't-go-wrong first meal of the day with the nutritional oomph to rev your sleepy engine and power you through the morning. It is composed of a balanced mix of low-glycemic carbohydrates, protein, and healthy fats that provides a slow, even-burning source of fuel that you won't suffer a sugar crash from. Foods low on the glycemic index (GI) release glucose gradually into the blood stream; examples include whole-grain and rye bread, fruit, lentils, soybeans, baked beans, and breakfast cereals based on wheat bran, barley, and oats. Foods high on the GI, which will quickly provoke high blood sugar levels, include refined flours such as pasta and white bread, potatoes, soft drinks, full-fat ice cream, chocolate bars, etc.

Given all that, a "power breakfast" might include a bowl of oatmeal with walnuts and berries, skim milk, and a teaspoon of brown sugar; a piece of whole-grain toast with almond or peanut butter; a cup of orange juice; and hot green tea or small coffee with milk.

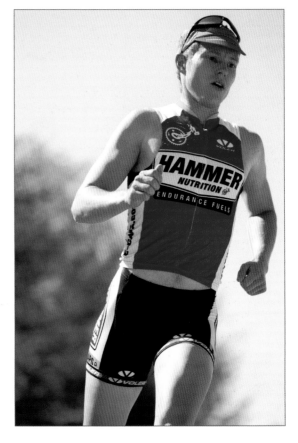

Sunday

- Training goal: One or more fast-paced walks of 10-plus minutes
- Nutrition goal: Eat a power break-fast
- In a notebook diary—your training journal—jot down notes about your walk and your breakfast. How long did you walk? What time did you go? How did you feel after the breakfast?
- Tip: "If you want to lose weight, start dieting at dinner, not breakfast. For example, eating a meager bowl

of Special K will increase your hunger and sweet cravings later in the day. A bigger breakfast (e.g., cereal, toast and peanut butter) can prevent afternoon or evening cookie binges. An adequate (i.e., 500- to 700-calorie) breakfast provides enough energy to enjoy exercise, instead of dragging yourself through an afternoon workout that feels like punishment." —Nutritionist and author Nancy Clark

Monday
- Training goal: One or more walks of 10-plus minutes
- Nutrition goal: Eat a power breakfast
- Spend ten minutes recording how the day went in your training journal
- Tip: Begin to make a habit of preparing your workout equipment the night before rather than waiting until the morning. Your shoes, your workout clothes, sunglasses, hat—any key equipment should be set out in an orderly way or packed into your gym bag. Making this a daily ritual will help you set a groove for your daily workout. If the mornings are a busy time for you, it will also help prevent forgetting something that could kill a workout.

Tuesday
- Training goal: Walk of 20-plus minutes
- Nutrition goal: Eat a power breakfast
- Journal
- Tip: As your walks get longer (and eventually evolve into walk/runs), you will want to experiment with layered clothing. Layers of jackets, long-sleeve shirts, sweatshirts, gloves, and hats—start out with as much as you need to be warm, and as your body continues to get warmer as you go, shed layers.

Wednesday
- Training goal: Go for one or more walks of 10 minutes or more
- Nutrition goal: Eat a power breakfast
- Journal
- Tip: Make sure your power breakfast includes slow-burning carbohydrates (oatmeal for example), fruit (a banana, an apple, or blueberries are good ones), and protein (a piece of whole grain toast with almond butter, for example). The mix of healthy carbs, protein, and fat will provide you a solid base of energy without any sugar rush or sugar crash. If you haven't been eating breakfast, you will love the way this makes you feel. Starting the day like this will help prevent cravings that might otherwise drive you into the never-ending cycle of junk food.

Thursday
- Training goal: Walk of 20-plus minutes
- Nutrition goal: Eat a power breakfast

- Journal
- Tip: Watch the documentary *Super Size Me*. Morgan Spurlock does an excellent job of showing how the fix of a fast-food meal leads to a vicious cycle of cravings and massive, nutritionally-challenged calorie intakes.

Friday
- Training goal: Walk of 20-plus minutes
- Nutrition goal: Eat a power breakfast
- Journal
- Tip: Beware the carb-only breakfast. Just a bowl of cereal will spike your blood sugar level and will eventually plummet, taking you with it. Once at the bottom of the plunge, you may find yourself crawling to the vending machine for a candy bar out of sheer desperation.

Saturday
- Training goal: Walk of 30-plus minutes
- Nutrition goal: Eat a power breakfast
- Journal
- Tip: The time for your workout is your time. If you're busy tending to a job or to family or both, make the time you spend training your personal time for you.

Week 2

Objectives:

1. Increase your walks to 30 minutes or more a day while you continue to adapt to the stress of daily exercise. In this week you will also add spurts of running.
2. In addition to your new power breakfast routine, this week you will work on consuming five to nine servings of fruit and vegetables a day. Americans get on average only two servings a day, and the fact is that a diet rich with fruit and vegetable consumption can help prevent heart disease and stroke, control blood pressure and cholesterol, and even prevent against the degeneration of cataracts. Of the many positive habits you can build into your diet, this is surely one of the best. Starting this week, strive to consume about five cups worth of fruits and vegetables each day. This roughly equates to nine servings. Vegetable and fruit salads, fruit smoothies, and sides of vegetables are simple ways to make good on this commitment. Since this new discipline alone will make huge changes in your health and how you feel, be sure to have fun with it. Venture outside of the box. Try out a variety of fruits and vegetables and constantly mix it up.
3. Continue to record your efforts in a daily journal

Sunday
- Training goal: Walk 20-plus minutes
- Nutrition goal: Five cups of fruits and vegetables

- Journal
- Tip: Take steps to eat out less and less. Bringing your lunch to work is a great start. When you go out, you're at the mercy of a hungry stomach and plentiful high-fat, high-calorie choices. Also, brown-bagging saves lots of money over time.

Monday
- Training goal: Walk 25 minutes or more. Include three one-minute runs.
- Nutrition goal: Five cups of fruits and vegetables
- Journal
- Tip: If you drink alcohol, start to think about refraining from anything more than one glass of wine or a beer a night. A glass of red wine each day may produce a healthy benefit—reducing the risk of heart disease. But anything over that often produces health problems.

Tuesday
- Training goal: Walk 30 minutes or more
- Nutrition goal: Five cups of fruits and vegetables
- Journal
- Tip: Make blueberries one of your choices for fresh fruit. "Blueberries are literally bursting with nutrients and flavor, yet very low in calories. Recently, researchers at Tufts University analyzed sixty fruits and vegetables for their antioxidant capability. Blueberries came out on top, rating highest in their capacity to destroy free radicals." —George Mateljan, *The World's Healthiest Foods*

Wednesday
- Training goal: Walk 30 minutes or more. Include four one-minute runs.
- Nutrition goal: Five cups of fruits and vegetables
- Journal
- Tip: A fantastic source of information is a website published by the Centers for Disease Control and Prevention, www.FruitsandVeggiesMatter.gov. You can plug in your numbers and get an idea of specifically what you should shoot for. According to the website, "Fruits and vegetables contain essential vitamins, minerals, and fiber that may help protect you from chronic diseases. Compared with people who consume a diet with only small amounts of fruits and vegetables, those who eat more generous amounts as part of a healthful diet are likely to have reduced risk of chronic diseases, including stroke and perhaps other cardiovascular diseases, and certain cancers."

Thursday
- Training goal: Walk 30 minutes or more
- Nutrition goal: Five cups of fruits and vegetables
- Journal

- Tip: The CDC website mentioned previously also has great information on how increasing your fruit and vegetable intake can help you lose weight. Here's a sample tip: "Substitute vegetables such as lettuce, tomatoes, cucumbers, or onions for 2 ounces of the cheese and 2 ounces of the meat in your sandwich, wrap, or burrito. The new version will fill you up with fewer calories than the original."

Friday
- Training goal: Walk 30 minutes or more. Include three two-minute runs.
- Nutrition goal: Five cups of fruits and vegetables
- Journal
- Tip: Right now, you're being asked to perform your exercise session daily. Considering that walking is low-impact and low-intensity, you can safely and effectively execute the session every day. Ideally, you will begin to seek ways in which to substitute walking for more sedentary choices, such as driving to run errands you could do walking. When we begin training at higher intensity levels and more demanding training routines, we will build in rest days. But altering your behavior so that you simply burn more calories throughout the day by moving around should become a daily practice for you.

Saturday
- Training goal: Walk for 40 minutes or more. Include one five-minute run.
- Nutrition goal: Five cups of fruits and vegetables
- Journal
- Tip: Take some time today to locate a nearby running or triathlon store. If you can find one, drop in and look around. Check for resources, local triathlon clubs, and local races. Running, cycling, and triathlon shops may be hubs of your endurance sports community.

Week 3

Objectives:
1. Add a bike ride into your regular walking and walk/run sessions.
2. As you continue to establish a power breakfast and increased fruit consumption habit, you will work toward improving your lunches and snacks.
3. Continue recording your progress in your journal.

Sunday
- Training goal: 30-minute walk/run. Start with 10 minutes of walking. For the second 10 minutes, alternate one minute of walking with one minute of running. Walk the final 10 minutes.

- Nutrition goal: Between breakfast and lunch, have a snack consisting of an apple and a piece of string cheese.
- Journal
- Tip: Wear a heart rate monitor for your exercise sessions, and record the heart rates you establish in your journal.

Monday
- Training goal: 30-minute walk
- Nutrition goal: If you normally eat lunch out, bring your own home-packed lunch
- Journal
- Tip: Packing the lunch at home: Tupperware can help you transport leftovers from the night before to your lunch table the next day. Don't forget to pack some fruit and vegetables.

Tuesday
- Training goal: Go for an easy bike ride
- Nutrition goal: Again, eat a healthy, homemade lunch
- Tip: Always wear a helmet when you ride your bike. Be sure it fits properly and is strapped on snugly. Practice caution while riding on roads. Being on a bicycle amongst the cars and SUVs makes you about as vulnerable as you can imagine.

Wednesday
- Training goal: 30-minute walk
- Nutrition goal: Homemade lunch
- Journal
- Tip: Make water your beverage of choice. Avoid high-calorie drinks and sodas.

Thursday
- Training goal: 30-minute walk/run
- Nutrition goal: Homemade lunch
- Tip: If you're having any trouble getting out the door for your walk/run, consider talking a friend into joining you. Make an appointment of it. Training buddies are one of the best tools to keep consistent.

Friday
- Training goal: Day off. Optional: 30-minute walk.
- Nutrition goal: Homemade lunch
- Journal
- Tip: Taking the occasional day off is good for your body and your mind. This will become more important as the intensity of your exercise sessions increases.

Saturday
- Training goal: 30-minute walk/run. Same as on Thursday.
- Nutrition goal: Have lunch out today if you like. Once a week is not going to hurt you. We recommend places like Subway that have clear information about ensuring a low-fat meal. Get into the habit of reading the nutritional postings at restaurants when they are available.

Week 4

Objectives:

1. Last week you walked, ran, and biked. This week you'll also get in the pool.
2. This week you will do your best to eat dinner on the early side.
3. Continue to journal.

Sunday
- Training goal: Enjoy a nice bike ride, 30 minutes or longer.
- Nutrition goal: Look up a recipe for dinner from the World's Healthiest Foods website, www.whfoods.org, and try something new.
- Journal
- Tip: I am the first to admit that I can't cook. However, as a student of the Trismarter .com folks, I've learned it's fun to become creative in meeting your nutritional needs with healthy, low-fat foods. Left to my own devices, I would create bland, boring (yet low-fat) dinners. After being advised by Rebecca Marks Rudy, a Trismarter.com nutritionist, I learned that contained within the pages of websites and magazines like *Cooking Light* there are indeed recipes that even I can tackle.

Monday
- Training goal: 30-minute walk/run. Include 10 minutes of continuous jogging.
- Nutrition goal: If you tend to eat dinner late (Rebecca Marks Rudy mentioned to me she has worked with clients who tend to eat dinner as late as 11 PM), trying pulling your dinnertime back a bit.
- Journal
- Tip: Try and wedge some time between when you eat dinner and when you hit the sack. You might find you'll sleep better, as you won't be digesting food when you're sleeping.

Tuesday
- Training goal: 30-minute walk
- Nutrition goal: Early dinner
- Journal
- Tip: Another good tip from Trismarter.com: Front load your primary meals with foods that have high water content. A small fruit or vegetable salad without heavy dressing,

for instance. The water content will be filling and you'll be less likely to eat more than a smart portion size when it comes time for the entrée.

Wednesday
- Training goal: Find a pool and check out the water. Work on getting comfortable (if you're not, read chapter 7 on swimming before you head to the pool) and try some easy, enjoyable laps. Your intention throughout your training for a first triathlon is to be relaxed and efficient in the pool (or lake or ocean). There's no need to emulate Mark Spitz.
- Nutrition goal: Early dinner
- Journal
- Tip: Part of being comfortable in the pool is a good pair of goggles that fits you well. If they leak or fog up, they'll drive you nuts. TYR, Speedo, and Aquasphere are good brands to try.

Thursday
- Training goal: 30-minute walk/run. Include a 10-minute stretch of jogging.
- Nutrition goal: Early dinner
- Journal
- Tip: Take a few minutes to stretch after your walk/run. Concentrate on your calves and hamstrings.

Friday
- Training goal: Take the day off. Optional: 30-minute walk.
- Nutrition goal: Early dinner
- Journal
- Tip: Pay attention to how you feel after eating a healthy, proportioned meal. Notice the energy you have.

Saturday
- Training goal: 40-minute walk/jog. Include 15 minutes of consecutive jogging.
- Nutrition goal: Early dinner
- Journal
- Tip: Congratulate yourself on completing

Week 5

You now have momentum with you. In weeks 5 and 6, you will schedule your training objectives to best fit your schedule. The 30-minute walks should be on the days you don't run, bike, or swim.

Objectives:

1. One swim: 30 minutes of easy, go-at-your-own-pace lap swimming
2. One 45-minute bike ride

3. One 40-minute walk/jog
4. Three walks, 30 minutes minimum

Nutrition goal for week 5: Add brown rice to your diet. Brown rice is a whole grain food that provides good energy, is loaded with fiber, and when mixed with beans, provides a complete protein. Have a cup of cooked brown rice at least twice this week as part of your lunch or dinner. Brown rice is the kind of staple that, if you rely on it every day, you will be all the better for it.

Week 6

The training in week 6 is the same as week 5. Guess what? You are living and training like a triathlete. It's this simple. If you're like most people, the feeling of improving your diet and including exercise throughout your week will energize you in such a way that you will declare, "I'm never going back to the way I was."

Objectives:

1. One swim: 30 minutes of easy, go-at-your-own pace lap swimming
2. One 45-minute bike ride
3. One 40-minute walk/jog. Try and jog the entire distance without stopping. Keep the pace slow and manageable.
4. Three 30-minute walks

Nutrition goal for week 5: Try out some healthy frozen dinners for various lunches and dinners. This is an optional addition to the enhancements you've made over the last five weeks. For someone with a busy, demanding lifestyle, having a frozen dinner, such as Lean Cuisine, waiting for you in the freezer after a long workday and commute can prevent you from picking up a pizza on the way home because you don't want to cook. Another tip from the Trismarter. com folks: One positive thing about a frozen dinner is portion control. It's built right in. The market for healthy, low-fat frozen dinners has exploded, and at your grocery store you can usually find an incredible selection.

That completes the six-week Basic Training program. If you've knocked it out, congratulations! You've made a huge step in your triathlon career. Now comes the fun part. It's time to target and prepare for your first race.

7
SWIMMING TUTORIAL

HOW TO TURN ROUGH WATERS INTO A SAFE, STRESS-FREE PLEASURE CRUISE

Let's face it, if you get tired cycling, you can coast or get off the bike. You could crash, but a very high percentage of bike crashes see the athlete walk away—very few threaten life. When running, you can always walk or stop. But you cannot stop completely during a swim. Drowning, as remote an event as it is, makes swimming arguably the most dangerous event in triathlon. Therefore, a healthy respect for swimming is important. Fear, however, takes that respect too far and should be addressed.

>—Steve Tarpinian, triathlon coach and author of *The Essential Swimmer.*

Except for those fortunate enough to have been on competitive swimming teams during their school years, most of us aspiring to be triathletes consider the swim to be the most difficult element to tackle.

When it comes to swimming, technique is almost everything. Right now I'm going to share with you a secret about training for the swim that could save you weeks, months, and years on the well-beaten path most take in their triathlon careers.

Here it is: Unlike running and cycling, going out and swimming so hard that your heart feels like it's going to burst is probably the biggest waste of time for an unskilled swimmer. Through sheer effort, a person can immediately begin making vast improvements in running and cycling by simply doing lots of biking and lots of running. Technique is valuable to both disciplines, but not necessary to making solid improvements in terms of endurance.

Swimming is a different animal. To quote Terry Laughlin, head coach of Total Immersion swimming, "If you try to improve by swimming more and harder—an approach that comes naturally for runners and cyclists—you'll mainly make your 'struggling skills' more permanent."

If you're training under Laughlin and he sees you doing anything that isn't fundamentally calm and relaxing, he's probably going to stop you and set you on a different path. The goal, Laughlin advises, is to become efficient in the water and to move through it in a "fish-like" manner. In his book, *Triathlon Swimming Made Easy* (isn't that a wonderful title?), Laughlin suggests adopting the following mandates:

1. Become your own swimming coach.
2. Practice mindfully, patiently, and intelligently.

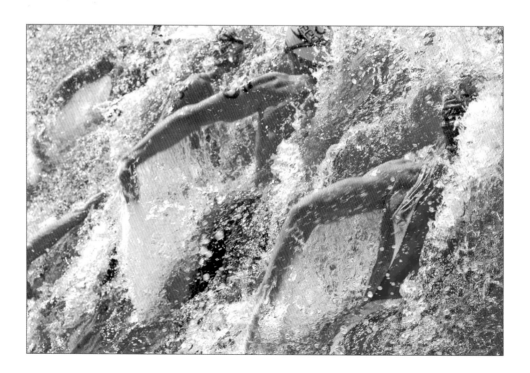

And for triathletes attending his workshops, Laughlin writes, "The most important message... is this: Your primary goal is not to swim faster. Focus first on swimming easier, and let speed be a natural product of your increased efficiency."

As I mentioned early in this book, I was a perfect candidate for Laughlin's approach. Previous to attending his workshop, I had tried the more common routes: Rigorous lap swimming, for one. I'd also consulted with personal trainers and I'd tried a few swim teams. I had been offered plenty of advice, but usually it simply short-circuited my brain. While I clung to the gutter at the pool's edge, a well-meaning personal trainer or coach would give me a laundry list of corrections to make: corrections to my position, the way my hands moved, my kick, and on and on and on. I'd throw myself into another lap, during which I would play a game of Whack-a-Mole with all the various flaws in my swimming. I'd be thinking about the position of my head or bilateral breathing, during which everything else fell apart, trying to drag me to the bottom. When no meaningful amount of progress resulted despite all of the pain and torture I was experiencing, it was difficult to keep coming back to the pool.

With that in mind, it is with some reluctance that I will attempt to coach you with your swimming from the pages of this book. I will try to pass on some basics that I learned from renowned instructors such as Laughlin and Steve Tarpinian; if you can attend a workshop given by either, do it. A highly regarded swim coach in your local area with a reputation of working wonders with beginners would also be a good start. If you prefer to do it yourself, both Laughlin and Tarpinian have videos and books. Per Terry's advice, you should think of yourself as your own swimming coach, and there are plenty of tools out there to help you do the job.

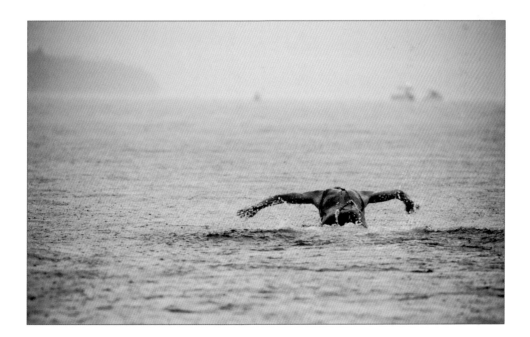

No matter what you do, don't stress out over the swim. Keep in mind that the length of the swim leg in a sprint triathlon, where most beginners literally get their feet wet in the sport, is only 400 yards. Even if you have to sidestroke or dog paddle your way through it, by completing the 12-week training program in chapter 11 you will succeed. No book or race will turn you into a hotshot triathlete overnight. But by entering and finishing that first short-distance sprint tri, you'll enter the world of thinking and living like an athlete. You will make it through the swim leg, breathe a sigh of relief, and go on to bike and run your way to the finish. It doesn't matter how fast you do the swim.

The goals for the swim leg in completing your first triathlon are as follows:

1. Be safe.
2. Finish the leg within any sort of time limit.
3. Use the least amount of energy necessary to compete goals one and two.

Being Safe

For obvious reasons, safety is the most important objective. Being safe in a triathlon requires that you have a doctor's seal of approval before even beginning to train for the sport. Specifically, we're talking about heart condition. I've covered the sport of triathlon for nearly 13 years, and there have been a small number of tragic deaths during that time. In many cases, the problem occurred as a heart attack during the swim leg.

I'm not a doctor, but having raced in triathlons for nearly 25 years, it seems logical to me that the nature of swimming itself and of racing in a swim pack—with all of the noise, excitement, and adrenaline that can manifest—is not a safe place for someone who has not executed a basic training program, is not physically fit, and/or is in a condition in which a heart attack could possibly take place.

If you've ever watched the Hawaii Ironman on TV, you have no doubt seen the spectacular image of 1,800 triathletes dashing off into the sea at the sound of a cannon. Some call it a "washing machine," which I've always felt is an apt description. It's thrilling to see. The idea of being in the middle of it is beyond thrilling. Now, most triathlons are not of this size and scope, and many triathlons around the country use what is called a wave start, where triathletes, grouped according to age, take off in smaller bursts rather than everyone going all at once. Still, it can be an intimidating situation for the weak swimmers. You'll still be swimming in open water and in range of other swimmers. If you choose, you can be right in the middle of it all when it starts.

So, since you know going in that the start of a triathlon can be overly stimulating, take steps to tone it all down a bit. First, have your doctor thoroughly check you out, letting him or her know you intend to participate in a triathlon. Two, execute a simple, thorough training program to prepare your body for the work involved in racing. And three, take steps at the race to minimize the craziness of the swim.

Turning the Swim from a Washing Machine into a Pleasure Cruise

I have participated in the Hawaii Ironman exactly one time, in the year 2000. I was competing as a lottery entrant, meaning that just about everyone else in the race (except for the other lottery contestants) was a much stronger swimmer than I. Yet I may have enjoyed one of the most peaceful swims of anyone that day. How? During the start, I was the ultimate gentleman and let everyone go ahead of me. I let the typhoon pass in front of me before I adjusted my goggles and started grinding through the water. So I sacrificed a few minutes right off the bat. But look at what I gained: I wasn't getting kicked in the face or elbowed in the gut by the dozens of people that would have been swimming over me. I had plenty of space in which to actually enjoy swimming in the Kailua Bay, and I generally expended far less energy than if I had tried to fight my way through the beast. I exited the water happy and alive, not exhausted, and went on to finish the race. The swim was certainly the easiest part of my day.

Hence my advice for your first triathlon: Sacrifice whatever straight line might exist on the swim course by swimming in the rear or to the outside of where the main group is swimming. This tactic will help assure that you make it through the day safely.

Finish the Leg Within the Time Limit

When researching or entering your race, note whether or not the race has a cutoff time for the swim. Tri-for-fun and sprint-distance races usually don't, but check their policy in terms of whether or not there is time limit for the swim finish.

If you're afraid you might be the last one out of the water, free yourself from this concern. Even if it turns out to be true, the spirit of triathlon is different than anything you might have experienced, for example, in grade-school sports. The last one out of the water in a triathlon— or across the finish line, for that matter—gets just as much applause, if not more, than the athlete first across the line. So the slower you are, the more likely you are to get a hero's welcome. Being a slow swimmer is nothing to be worried about.

Using the Least Amount of Energy Possible

You may have watched Olympic swimming events. Except for some of the distance events, most Olympic competition is high-speed sprint racing. Triathlon swimming is different in a number of respects. First, an Olympic swimmer doesn't have to climb out of the pool at the end of the race to race on a bike or run; a triathlete does. For that reason alone, it's essential that you don't blow all of your energy on the swim.

The aquatic environment introduces several critical variables that can produce struggle for a human being. Poor form and position produce tremendous resistance, and if you go gangbusters trying to increase your speed, your muscles will fill with lactic acid and you'll get no satisfying return on your investment. Breathing is another big problem. If you haven't been swimming in years, your first sessions of lap swimming in the pool can trigger something that feels more like hyperventilation than breathing. I know this because I've experienced it. In the program presented within these pages, you will go to the pool and use the stroke you're most comfortable with and slowly, easily work your way into finding the right rhythms so that you can breathe deeply and easily, and keep the lactic acid—and panic in general—at a minimum. If you need to use the sidestroke, backstroke, or dog paddle, this is what you'll do. Once you've finished your first triathlon and earned the right to be called a triathlete, well, then you can develop a freestyle stroke that moves you along a little faster.

TECHNIQUE TUTORIAL, PART 1:
GET AQUA-COMFORTABLE

Few are better than Terry Laughlin at teaching non-swimmers how to swim and frustrated veteran swimmers how to swim faster. All are grateful, but beginners particularly so, because their new skill opens up a whole new sport for them. But before we get to his method, however, we must address the true water-wary, those who freak out at the very idea of getting into water above knee level. For them, getting comfortable in water over your head is necessary before you start to formally learn how to swim. If you are not at that point, have no fear. Steve Tarpinian of www.SwimPower.com offers the following fail-safe recommendations:

1. **First, learn how to tread water.**
   "The basic technique for treading water is to sweep the arms in and out, creating a sculling motion, which creates lift and easily keeps your head above water," Tarpinian says. An eggbeater or scissor-style kick can be added so as to make the arm movement even easier.

   Tarpinian says that treading water can usually be learned in a few practice sessions. "There is a big boost of confidence that comes with knowing that no matter what happens, you can stop swimming and tread water with minimal effort," he adds.

2. **Get comfortable with your breathing.**
   If your breathing isn't relaxed and efficient, Tarpinian says you will always struggle and be tense in the water. "Getting oxygen is part of the process of creating energy in the muscles," he explains. "You would not get too far without breathing when you run, and you won't get far with limited or no oxygen in your muscles while you swim."

   To practice how to take a breath, go to the side of the pool, strap your goggles on, lean over, put your face in the water, and roll it from side to side. Then, holding onto the coping with one hand, try it with your body extended into a full horizontal position.

   "Try taking five breaths on each side (right and left) and really taking your time," says Tarpinian. "Breathe out when your face is in the water and roll your body to the side and breathe in when your mouth is out of the water. Use the guideline of one goggle in the water and one out to be sure you have your head in the correct position."

Being comfortable in the water is the first and most important step toward safely and confidently completing the swim leg in a triathlon. Once you have accomplished this, you can begin to work on working on a smooth, efficient stroke. For that, we go to Terry Laughlin.

TECHNIQUE TUTORIAL, PART 2:
HOW TO "SWIM LIKE A FISH"

You've heard of the old saying, "Different strokes for different folks." The key to Laughlin's approach is "Less strokes for all folks."

Laughlin loves to tell the story of how, to get faster back in college, he pinwheeled his arms faster and faster—and all it did was wear him out. He soon came to realize, after looking at a tape of great swimmers, like Russia's Alexander Popov, that the key to great swimming was not more and faster strokes, but getting more out of every stroke. And that required a radical rejiggering of his form and his thinking.

First and foremost, remember this, says Laughlin: Water is roughly a thousand times denser than air, and thus is a hugely difficult medium to move through. Because of this, generating more force in order to move faster through the water is a poor strategy. A more effective strategy is to make your body form more "hydrodynamic"—more streamlined, or able to cut through the water with less drag. He calls it "fish-like swimming."

That literally means to adopt the profile of a fish. Instead of plowing through the water like a flat-bottomed barge, cut through it with the narrow keel of yacht. Doing so allows you to take fewer strokes.

For the techies among us, Laughlin likes to illustrate his concept with the equation "$V = SL \times SR$," where V is velocity, SL is stroke length, and SR is the stroke rate. He advises this equation because increasing velocity by favoring stroke rate is risky. That's because as you increase your stroke rate to achieve more speed, your stroke length gets shorter. On top of that, you get more tired. That's because shorter strokes mean that you are flat-bottomed like a barge for a greater percentage of the time. By contrast, when your arms are extended in a long stroke, you are tilted longer on your side, like a boat keel, slicing through the H_2O more efficiently.

The upshot: As your arms move faster, it requires greater and greater amounts of energy to move shorter and shorter distances. Ultimately, even if you could achieve super stroke rate, you would run out of gas.

This is an especially ill-advised idea in the sport of triathlon. Since triathletes have two other sports to go after the swim, the rapid-stroke-rate strategy would probably have negative results. You'd have expended a lot of valuable energy in the water that would have better been saved for the bike and the run. This is hugely inefficient because you can make up huge chunks of time on the bike and run compared to the swim. Bottom line: moving your arms like a madman might result in minimal gain on the swim, but cause maximal loss on the next two events.

By clearing your mind of the need for arm speed, Laughlin opens you up to the idea of focusing on how your body is positioned in the water at each moment. He beats you over the head with the concept of looking at swimming as a technique sport, similar to the way people think about golf and tennis. He begs you: Do not look at swimming as a strength sport, like running or cycling.

I can't teach you on paper the way that Laughlin can, and certainly can't give you the epiphany you'd get in one of his weekend clinics. But as I see it, and as I have used it in my own experience, there are just a few easy-to-understand technical concepts that will help you reap the majority of the benefits of Laughlin's Total Immersion philosophy. Here's what has worked for me:

1. **Think hydrodynamics:** Freeze a sleek, blade-like image in your mind. Visualize the body as a fast-moving aqua vessel—like a fish—moving through water, creating as little drag as possible. If you think of a ship, think yacht, not barge.

2. **Get comfortable being on your side:** Do drills that teach you how to extend the period of time that your body is tipped on your hip—vertically. At his clinic, we literally spent hours laying on our sides in the water, floating with one arm extended. This literally is the "fish-like" position he talks about.

3. **Now, glide:** Fight the urge to surge. Keep your hand out in front, like the bow of a ship, helping you ride the momentum of the stroke from the other hand as long as possible. Before you begin rotating the body and pulling the hand back to grab water, get big distance from every stroke. In our clinic, Laughlin made a big deal of counting our "before" and "after" strokes, and showing us how many fewer strokes it took to get across the pool—often at an faster pace, especially for the poorer swimmers. Above all, remember this: less strokes equal less work. And more fun.

4. **Swim downhill:** "Swimming downhill" is a Laughlin catchphrase that I can't get out of my mind. It refers to keeping your body slightly hinged at the waist. That position will help keep you from sinking by getting air, which wants to rise, deeper into your lungs, effectively floating you like a buoy. When you are sideways, it doesn't matter as much. But on the brief intermediate stage between the right and left arm extensions, this slight "downhill" orientation better floats your boat.

Bottom line: It is quite possible to reconfigure your body in the water to make swimming an enjoyable activity that you even begin to look forward to. If you practice a few simple principles long enough to make them habit, you will soon be able to glide effortlessly through the water, instead of being dragged down by it.

When you get to that point, as I have, you will find that you can achieve a beatific endorphin high that is strikingly similar to the runner's high that we all love.

SPECIAL ADVANCED SWIMMING SECTION

You know what comes after you get up to speed: you want more of it. I think the best way to get it is, once more, to listen to Terry Laughlin. Not surprisingly, he pushes "ease" over "effort," emphasizing mechanical efficiency to cover more distance with fewer strokes.

Ease Your Way into a Faster 1500

Laughlin's tips on improving your time in the metric mile—the 1500-meter swim—won't strike you as much different from the basics that he teaches to beginners. "The natural inclination is to think, 'I need to swim faster workouts to swim faster in the race,'" he says. But, of course, he proves this assumption wrong. "A much more promising way to improve your 1500," he says, "is by seeking more ease, rather than more effort."

Laughlin backs his "easy does it" argument with stats from USA Swimming. They show that the world's best 1500-meter swimmers—men who swim it in less than 15 minutes and women who do it in sub-16 minutes—are just 9 percent mechanically efficient. Over 90 percent of their energy is consumed by making waves and pushing water out of the way.

"If elite swimmers lose 90 percent of their energy to wave making, I'd guess that the average triathlete might be about 5 percent mechanically efficient," says Laughlin. His math shows that improving to just 6 percent is a 20 percent gain in efficiency—about what it takes to improve from 30 minutes to 25 minutes in 1500 meters.

Converting this to speed figures, Laughlin says that a 30-minute 1500 represents a pace of 2:00 per 100 meters, while a 25-minute finish represents an average of 1:40 per 100—still a relatively leisurely speed.

"The secret to 25 minutes isn't to kill yourself trying to go faster, especially considering the 50 kilometers of running and cycling that usually follow it," he says. "It's to learn to swim 1:40 with such ease that you can do it indefinitely without tiring.

Here's Laughlin's three-step plan for getting there:

1. **Take fewer strokes.** Virtually everyone who swims a sub-15 minute 1500 meters can swim lap after lap in a 25-yard pool in 12 or fewer strokes, at speeds most of us would find breathtaking. The average triathlete takes nearly twice that many strokes per length. If your average stroke count (i.e., what you can hold for an hour or so of repeats, not what you do for one careful length) is over 20, you need to reduce it to at least the high teens.

2. **Maintain a lower stroke count for longer.** Once you improve to a lower count, you can increase the distances you cover at that count with a simple exercise: If you're used to taking 20 strokes per lap, limit yourself to 17 or 18. Each passing lap requires more concentration on keeping your bodyline sleek and strokes effective.

   "Whenever I've decided to focus on increasing my stroke length, I swam slower," says Laughlin. "So I paid less attention to the clock and more to the details of my stroke. As my nervous system adapted, I gradually regained the lost speed, but spent less energy for it."

   Practice at short distances—25, 50, 75, 100 yards. If your stroke count goes above your targets (say 17 or 18 per lap), Laughlin says to do one or more of the following: (a) slow down, (b) increase your rest to four or five yoga breaths, or (c) swim more quietly. When you can successfully complete the set in your new stroke count, double the distance.

   "Going *further* with that count is more important than going *faster* with it," says Laughlin.

   When you successfully complete that set in the same stroke count, he says go for an entire swim, say 1000 yards. Keep the new stroke count without straining or exaggerated push offs. "If you start taking more strokes, say 19, your next lap is super-slow drilling, then three deep breaths and begin swimming again," says Laughlin. Over time, your drills will turn into straight swimming—longer *efficient* swimming.

3. **Add strokes back in.** When 17 strokes per lap (or whichever count you're working at) becomes your new normal, you can then go faster by adding one smooth stroke.

"This turns descending sets into coordination exercises, rather than tests of your intestinal fortitude," says Laughlin. For example, he explains, on a set of 15 × 100, swim five rounds of three, the first 100 in each round in a total of 68 strokes (average of 17 strokes per lane), the second at 72 strokes (average of 18 stokes per lane) and the third at 76 strokes. On each succeeding round you aim to swim more smoothly at each count, to transition more seamlessly from one count to the next and to gain materially in speed each time you *choose* to increase your stroke count. Adjust the stroke counts in the example to suit your own stroke count, as developed in step 2.

Go for the Flow

Laughlin doesn't advocate "no pain no gain."

"I coached an Olympic medalist and American record holder while he was a young age grouper," he says. "When I asked him how his record-breaking races felt, he told me they were the easiest he'd ever swum. Four world-record holders described the same experience. My best races have likewise involved no pain, just a wonderful sense of being in command."

Bottom line: Great swimming virtually always happens in a "flow state," not a haze of pain, which is even more important when you have to cycle and run at your best after swimming. Put most of your focus on doing whatever it takes to feel better. Whatever feels good is good.

OPEN-WATER TRAINING IN THE POOL

No ocean or lake to swim in? Work on open-water skills in your pool, says Tim Crowley, CSCS, PES, a coach at Carmichael Training Systems. Just follow some of the drills and training sets below.

Drills

Eyes-closed swimming: To learn how to swim straight (a common problem in open water) without relying on a black line, close your eyes and swim 25 yards in an empty lane with your eyes shut. If you bump into the lane lines, you are not swimming straight. You can also get the effect by closing your eyes when facing down but opening them when you turn to breathe.

Drafting: With two or three swimmers, create a pace line, switching leaders every 25 or 50 meters as the leader pulls off to the side and then sprints to the back of the pace line.

Close quarters: Swim with two to three swimmers shoulder-to-shoulder across the lane. This simulates swimming in a pack. Alternate the swimmer in the middle.

Buoy turning: Place a sturdy floating object at the end of the lane to practice turning a buoy without using the wall. This drill can be combined with the close-quarters drill by racing down the lane and around the buoy, offering fun competition as well.

Starts

An advantage on race day is getting out in front fast, which helps you avoid the start-line mob scene and calmly settle into your pace more quickly.

Deep-water start: Tread water in the deep end, then sprint without using the wall.

Getting out fast: Bolting into clear water fast allows you to settle into your goal pace faster and draft off faster groups, but it hits you with a surge of lactic acid. To teach your body to assimilate, do intervals four to six weeks before the race. Do repeats of 200 to 400 meters, hammering out the first 100 meters, then settling into race pace for the remainder of the set. You will quickly find out if you went out too hard.

Over/under intervals: Increasing your pace above threshold is necessary at the start, catching up to a faster group to draft, approaching the exit or a buoy, and passing someone or a group. Over/under intervals, like the sets below, elevate your swim speed above lactate threshold, then train you to return to race pace without need for a prolonged recovery.

2-4 × 450 meters (100m race pace, 50m slightly faster. Repeat three times, continuously)

2-4 × 500 meters (25m race pace, 25m fast, 50m race pace, 50m fast, 75m race pace, 75m fast, 100m race pace, 100m fast)

Sighting

Go off course and you'll be beaten out of the water by slower but more experienced open-water swimmers who can navigate. Do these two drills to stay on target.

Sighting while breathing: On longer swim sets, take a breath, turn your head forward with your eyes just above water level, and focus on an object at the far end of the pool. Done as a fluid motion once or twice each length, it'll get you comfortable with sighting without disrupting your swim tempo.

Heads-up swimming: A common lifeguard skill, heads-up swimming can prove invaluable in a crowded swim start, or in rough water where sighting buoys may be difficult. Swimming a length with your head and shoulders up forces you to kick harder and requires more energy. Do 50-meter repeats with the first 25 heads-up.

LEARNING THE FLIP TURN

According to coaches Trip Hedrick and Clark Campbell, the flip turn is an essential part of your swim workouts, keeping you in the flow and adding a fun, competitive edge to your workout regimen. Also it's a fun "free ride" that makes you feel like you know what you're doing.

There are three steps to a flip turn: (1) the somersault/flip to a foot plant on the wall, (2) a streamline push-off, (3) a twist onto the stomach transitioning into the freestyle stroke. Below, the rules to master them. For more details, check the Triathlete Technique and Training series at www.ChampionshipProductions.com.

The somersault

Approach the flip while keeping the shoulders parallel to the surface of the water without twisting. To practice it, follow this progression:

1. **Jumping somersault:** Go to chest-deep water and assume a standing at attention position. Jump forward, sliding your chest over the water, and execute a chin-to-chest, shoulders-to-thighs, and heels-to-butt somersault, keeping your hands at your side throughout. Try to feel your calves and heels slapping the water as you finish your spin.

2. **Hand-to-hand partner drill:** With a partner standing behind you with arms out and palms up, extend your arms back, placing your palms down on his or hers. Lower yourself to neck level in the water, drop your chin and execute a somersault, maintaining hand-to-hand contact throughout to keep shoulders even.

3. **Mid-pool somersault with strokes:** After three strokes, position both hands at your side, take three to four kicks to flatten the shoulders on the water, then do a somersault.

4. **Don't lift the head:** A common mistake is the momentum-killing tendency to lift the head to spot the wall, which lowers the hips and wrecks the flip. To stop this, keep an eye on the line where the bottom of the pool and the wall meet and don't breath on the last two strokes.

5. **Flip turn with streamline push-off on the back:** Swim into the wall, somersault, plant the feet, extend the hands into a streamline position and push off onto the back holding the streamline. A non-horizontal push-off probably means you're over-rotating; stop this by lifting chin off chest as the heels come over the water towards the butt.

6. **Flip turn with streamline transition into freestyle:** *To get that on-your-side position off the wall, simply angle your toes to the side you are most comfortable pushing off on. Be careful not to twist the body to that direction.*

7. **The streamline:** Streamlining is estabishing a low-resistance body position that maximizes wall speed. Get it by narrowing yourself, drawing everything closer to the mid-line of the body, squeezing the ears with the biceps, and squeezing the hips. Don't overreach, which causes tremendous curve in the lower back as the ribs flare outward.

8
CYCLING
TUTORIAL

HOW TO TAKE ADVANTAGE OF TRIATHLON'S LONGEST LEG

Like most American kids, the best birthday present ever was my first bike. It was as close as you could get to flying. I remember the first time I went on a long bike ride—about 40 miles in a single day—when I was about 14. I was a mess at the end of it, and the mistakes I made were classic of anyone getting into road riding or touring without heeding the basic tips.

The first and foremost tip when it comes to taking up cycling is comfort. This was a key point made by six-time Hawaii Ironman champion Dave Scott in his book, *Dave Scott's Triathlon Training,* written back in 1986. Scott hailed from a water-polo background, so cycling was completely new to him. Like many runners and swimmers first getting on the bike to train, the thought of expensive clothing (and cycling clothing is expensive) seems an exotic excess. In my first triathlon, in 1983, I rode my bike, both in training and in the race, with running shoes and running shorts. I hadn't learned the lesson from my ride as a 14-year-old, where by the end of the ride I was sore, sunburned, chafed, and completely beat. The same happened in my first triathlon, when I rode the 56-mile leg in running shorts. I made a tough day a dozen times tougher.

Dave learned this too and pointed it out in his book. A pair of cycling shorts with a chammy is worth its weight in gold. Cycling gloves, cycling socks, good cycling shoes, sunglasses, a proper jersey with pockets, and a comfortable helmet are necessities for longish rides.

Will you need this for your first sprint triathlon? No, you could certainly make it through a 12-mile bike leg or so without much damage, but trust me, your enjoyment of the training and of the race itself will make the investment pay off.

We covered what you need for this in your shopping spree, but it's important to understand why you're spending all this money for bike riding. In addition to comfortable gear, you'll need to be set up on your bike in a way that's relatively in tune with your body.

Once you have these matters covered, and are comfortable on your bike, you'll be able to relax and enjoy being outside burning up calories in what is certainly one of the most enjoyable forms of cardiovascular exercise around. If you've ever ridden a Lifecycle or other type of indoor bike

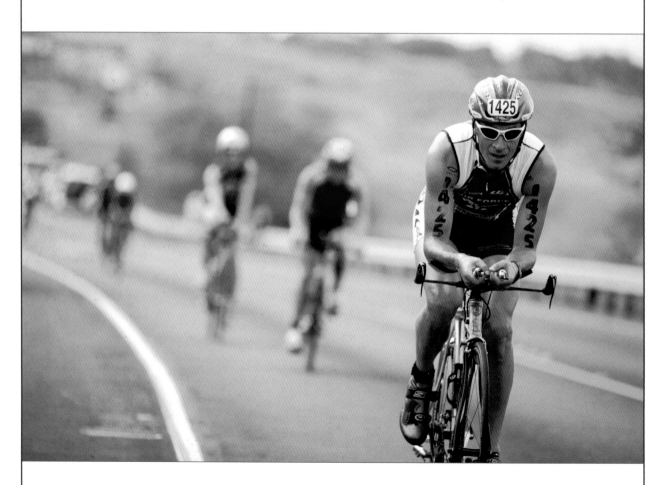

in a gym, you know that 20 minutes can seem like hours. If you find a good place in the park or the country to go riding, you'll notice an inverse effect: a couple of hours can go by very fast.

Cycling also offers the most sociable aspect to triathlon: the group ride. Across the country, triathlon and cycling clubs usually sponsor weekend rides, often for riders of all levels. Once you give this a try, you'll probably be hooked for life. Most bike riding is done at a pace where conversations can easily be held, especially when your goal is to finish races as opposed to win them. If you like to make friends and hang with buddies, rest assured that this is the spirit of many weekend group rides. To find out about local rides, your best source is your local biking or triathlon shop. Group rides are also a terrific place to learn basic bike-handling techniques, pack riding tips, and other essential skills.

Another favorable aspect of cycling is that, like running, it offers immediate improvement simply by getting out there and doing it. And as much as you can grow to love swimming and running, cycling probably offers the most fun of all three disciplines. Let's look into how to get started.

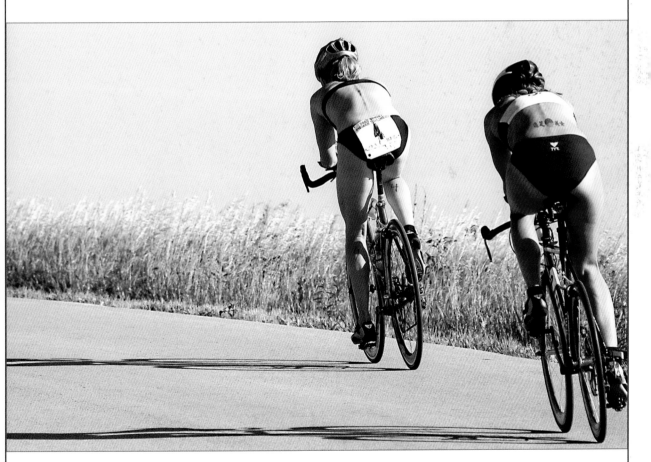

STEP 1: THE RIGHT FIT

Cycling's easy. Just hop on your bike and ride it, right? Wrong. First, you need to make sure it fits.

The rule is the same for beginners and veterans alike: Whether you ride a garage-sale Huffy ten-speed or a $7,000 carbon-titanium frame dream machine with aero wheels, make sure it fits. Just like a suit coat or a dress, a bike looks and feels best when it is properly fitted to your body. In fact, the fit of a rider's bicycle is arguably the most important equipment-related issue in triathlon. A proper fit not only makes you much more comfortable, powerful, aerodynamic, and faster on the bike, but leads to better bike-to-run transitions and a better run. No one is better at explaining why than Christopher Kautz, the owner of Bay Area–based PK Racing Technologies.

"A properly fitted triathlon bicycle is one that allows the athlete to be comfortable, maintain a neutral spine, generate good power, stabilize the bike and body, exchange air, take in

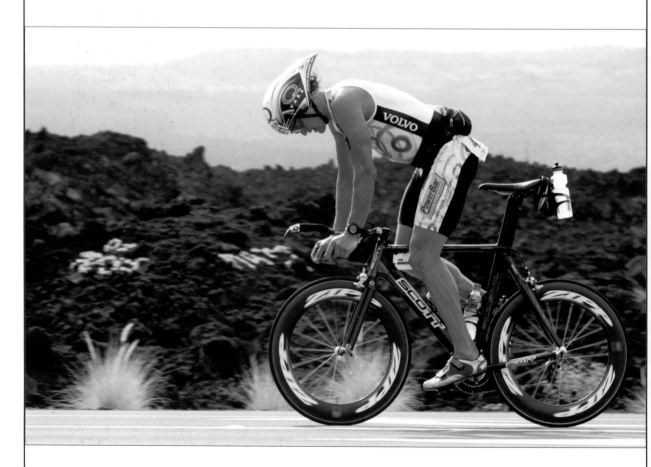

nutrients, cut through the air, pedal more efficiently, and transition well to running," says Kautz, who performs elaborate studies of each individual client's biomechanics, flexibility, and strength. "Bike fit is too often overlooked by athletes, and too often based upon myth and lore. It is essential to think of bike fitting in terms of kinetic chains."

I love the term "kinetic chain." I had no idea what it meant when I first heard it, but it's logical. An example of a kinetic chain, according to Kautz, is an athlete experiencing a sore left shoulder as a result of an improperly aligned right cleat. The improper cleat rotation will cause a misalignment of the leg, a subsequent rotation of the pelvis, leading to the athlete sitting crooked on the bike, resulting in a sore shoulder. So you get the idea of how one improperly placed or fitted individual component can affect you on a bike.

In fitting yourself to a bike, Kautz says to "sequence it from the ground up"—start with the shoes, go up to the seat, then finally adjust the handlebars.

Shoe Setup

Bike shoes support the arch and, with clipless pedals, transfer power. But no two systems are alike. Different cycling shoes and pedal systems have different sole thicknesses and stack heights, respectively, that in turn affect saddle height. Furthermore, moving the cleats fore and aft on the shoe affects relative length of the foot.

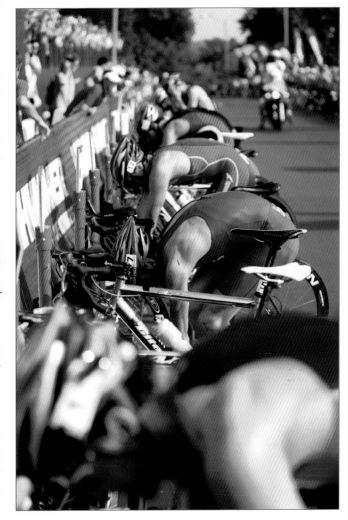

Kautz says that most athletes wear cycling shoes too short for their arches, placing the cleats too far back on the foot. The ball of the foot should be placed on the trailing edge of the pedal's axle.

By locating the cleat under the second metatarsal head, slightly further ahead than most people do, you gain mechanical advantage by lengthening the effective lever arm, which allows for more force production. The second metatarsal position also allows for more efficient acceleration of the pedal.

Saddle Position Setup

Don't sit with a posterior (or backward) tilt to the pelvis, as you do slumped in a chair, says Kautz. Proper cycling posture requires a slight forward tilt of the pelvis, so that the pressure from the saddle is just on the front edges of the sit bones, rather than straight under or on the back of them. The benefit: By rotating the pelvis forward it is possible to maintain a neutral spine, allowing for activation of the core muscles that provide a stable anchor for the rider and allow better power development and transfer.

By contrast, the posterior tilt of many bikers leads to low back flexion, which is bad news: it curves your lumbar spine into a C-shape, stretching out low back ligaments and risking low-back pain; it turns off the gluteal muscles, forcing the quads to work harder; and it crimps your digestion, lungs, and diaphragm, limiting deep breathing.

So how to adjust the saddle? Keep the nose level or minimally tilted (under 2 to 2.5 degrees from level in either direction) to provide a solid pedaling platform; keep the height at a point that allows for a comfortable extension of the leg without causing the athlete to overreach to the pedals. If it's set too low, you work too hard, putting excessive pressure on the front of the knee and inhibiting muscular recruitment. Conversely, a saddle set too high strains the hamstrings (which attach to the down-tilted pelvis). A saddle that is the right height will give you an ideal bend of between 145 and 155 degrees at the back of the knee.

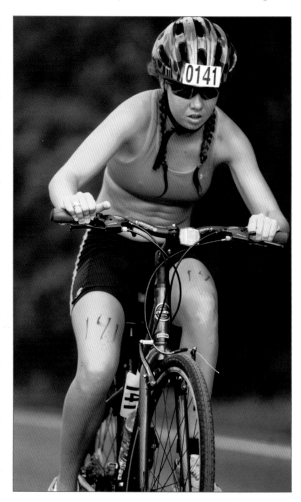

Aerobar and Handlebar Setup

Handlebar placement offers the most leeway in a bike fitting. They should be positioned to help you maintain good posture (neutral spine), and avoid over-reaching. The aerobar pads should be at a broad, comfortable width and allow stable handling, yet narrow enough to provide aerodynamic benefits. Handlebar height depends on how far back the saddle moves (the further back, the higher the bars need to be). Highly flexible athletes, particularly those with good hip flexion (the ability to bring the femur to the torso), can run lower handlebars and still maintain proper posture on the bike. Less flexible athletes will need the bars higher to maintain proper posture. Morphologically, a number of variables such as arm length, torso length, and leg length will affect how much room is available for drop to the bars. Lastly, race distance needs to be considered in order that the position be comfortable enough for the athlete to maintain.

Regarding aerobar fit and positioning, the elbows should be slightly in front of the shoulders in a vertical plane. You should rest on your bones, sparing your arm muscles; strain in neck and shoulders indicates you are reaching too far.

Dealing with Neck Pain

Speaking of pain in the neck, John Howard, three-time Olympic cyclist, 1981 Ironman winner, and esteemed triathlon school coach (www.JohnHowardSports.com) says perfect fit or not, you have to be prepared to deal with it. "The aero-position posture often severely contorts the body, with the first indication being neck pain," he says. "It places your head in a tilted-back posture in order to see the road. Muscles that are contracted like this for the duration of the ride produce muscle responses that cause all of the posterior neck muscles to shorten.

Solutions include raising the handlebars and massage/stretching. In the latter, you want to work the three key muscles along the skull line (occipital ridge)—the trapezius, splenius capitis, and splenius cervicis—which as a group laterally extend the neck, and rotate and tilt the head.

Here's some detail: Begin working both sides of your neck, systematically working one side with the opposite hand, then the other side. Place the fingers on the muscles just to the side of your cervical vertebrae. If you feel tightness, gently massage those neck muscles. Working from your skull down to your shoulder, start next to your spine, then about one inch to the side. Rub out tight muscles; your goal is to create a smooth muscle line. The action should include gradually increased pressure, working the belly of the muscle.

Stretching: To increase the stretch of the muscles, slowly drop your head toward your chest and slightly turn your chin to the opposite shoulder while holding the muscle. Hold the stretch ten to 15 seconds working up to 45 seconds. After the stretch, shake out your shoulders and neck. You can effectively work on the back of the neck muscles by using a 24-inch length of wooden dowel. Follow the picture, being very careful not to press directly on the vertebrae and only using enough strength to cause slight discomfort on the muscles. To enhance the movement, slowly drop your chin to your chest and draw your shoulders down while you are pressing the neck muscles. You can continue pressing the dowel all the way to your shoulder to release tension in the trapezius muscle.

STEP 2: PROPER SPIN: COME FULL CIRCLE

You never forget how to ride a bike, they say. But what if you never learned how to ride a bike correctly in the first place?

This may sound strange, but the truth is that most of us don't really know how to pedal a bike. We are mashers, pounding the pedals down like pistons in an engine, hammering our quadriceps muscles into oblivion. The quads, the big muscles on the front of the thigh, are the

100 percent go-to muscles for pedaling, right? Well, not exactly. Especially if you do what every cycling coach from Peoria to Perth will tell you: Pedal in circles.

Riders who have smoother and more circular pedal strokes at a relatively rapid cadence (80 to 100) can go longer and stronger. Triathletes who pedal circles have more left at the end of the day, more left for the run. And they also have lower incidences of injuries and comfort-related issues than riders with less balanced and slower strokes.

That's because riders who pedal efficient circles have more balanced muscle groups (thus reducing strain) and are more balanced in the saddle. A balanced stroke means that you are recruiting a variety of muscles throughout the entire range of the pedal circle. Want proof? Just look closely at one revolution of the pedals: Through the front of the stroke (centering at three o'clock) the primary muscles being used are the quadriceps. The front of the stroke is an area that most riders do not need to focus much attention on, as the quadriceps tend to work by default when riding a bike. That's why you need to focus on the bottom, back, and top of the stroke, where optimal muscle recruitment requires a more active technique.

One guy I've found who is very good at explaining this technique is Ian Buchanan, co-owner of Fit Werx, a triathlon and road cycling specialty shop in Waitsfield, Vermont (www .FitWerx.com): "Once you are through the front of the stroke and heading into the bottom of the stroke (about five o'clock), you want to start transferring muscle engagement in the upper leg from the quadriceps to the hamstrings," says Buchanan. "Entering the bottom of the stroke, focus on keeping your heel flat and pulling your foot through and back (as if you were wiping mud off the bottom of your foot). If done properly, you will feel the muscles around your shin engage as the transfer from the quadriceps to the hamstrings (pushing to pulling muscles) takes place. As you come around to the back of the stroke (from about seven o'clock on) focus on unweighting the foot by pulling your instep up against the top of your shoe with your calf and hamstrings. Many riders will lift their heel slightly at this point (known as ankling) to assist with fluidity of the stroke and active muscle engagement."

To complete the transition to the hamstrings successfully, Buchanan says that you want to make sure that your pelvis is tilted (rolled) forward on the saddle (sitting on your pelvic platform). "The easiest way I've found to describe this position is to have you think about your pelvic position when you are getting out of a chair. The hamstrings need to be at nearly a ninety-degree angle to the pelvis to fire effectively and lift us from the chair," he says. If you read the section on bike fit, above, this ought to sound familiar.

Once you are past the back of the stroke (around nine o'clock), the hamstrings are assisted by the glutes before the stroke enters another potential flat spot at the top (eleven to one o'clock) of the stroke. This area, by the way, is arguably the most difficult in which to maintain active muscle recruitment, because it requires use of the hard-to-activate hip flexor and psoas (core abdominal) muscles. To engage these muscles, push the instep of your foot into the tongue of the shoe, driving and pushing the pedal across the top of the stroke to help you keep momentum. Once through the top of the stroke, bring the foot back horizontal to the ground as you head back into the front of the stroke again with the quadriceps-based pushing muscles.

I know what you might be thinking right now: They've taken the simple pleasure of pedaling a bike and complicated it to the point where I'm worried. But don't stress out. I've found that having things to think about while swimming, running, and cycling actually makes the time go faster. You will, too.

For training, Buchanan recommends that you learn proper pedaling by focusing on one portion of your pedal stroke at a time. "Once you master the sections independently, it will be easier to integrate them," he says. "Also, expect it to feel like additional work at first and to require practice. You are asking muscles to fire in patterns they are not used to and they need to gain strength and familiarity with those demands before they will work optimally."

The payoff comes quickly. Pedaling efficient circles reduces the strain on everything, from the neck and shoulders to the lower back and butt, and allows you to ride significantly faster with the same amount of energy expenditure. And if you're stuck indoors during a cold winter snowstorm, consider yourself lucky. After all, it's an ideal time to work on your pedal circle.

STEP 3: LEARNING YOUR GEARS BEYOND THE BIG RING

Now that you know why you should pedal in circles and have learned the technique for doing it, the next step is to learn how to use your gear shifters.

Again, we all think we know how to shift gears. Climbing a hill? Downshift. Hammering on the flats? Shift it into the big ring. Easy, right? If you were just cruising the bike path for fun, you could stop right there. But if you want to be a triathlete, where every event by definition is a race, you want to learn how to go as fast as you can, and that will require more than rudimentary shifting knowledge. If you're gear-phobic, calm down. You are not dumber than anyone else. In fact, to hear cycling Hall of Famer John Howard tell it, *most* triathletes, including the elites, are slower than they need to be because they shove it in the big chain ring and leave it there.

"Most triathletes are underpowered on the bike—they can't maintain high output wattage," says Howard, "and that's because they are constantly training in the same gear without much variation in cadence."

It's a huge wasted opportunity, he explains. While most coaches are sticklers at defining zones, time, and distance, few seem to give much consideration to gear selection for maximizing training value.

Howard teaches his students that gains in cycling are achieved through a widely varied training program. "This can be done by starting every ride in the small chainring and gradually building the cadence up to the high nineties and into the hundreds," he says. "The first 30 minutes of every ride should include this low gear warm-up to condition the various energy systems, increasing blood flow and synovil fluid in the joints. This is especially important to multisport athletes who should be constantly striving to overlap training layers and achieve a harmonious transition between sports.

Howard recommends a "soft taper" from each hard workout. This includes dropping the gear in the closing 15 minutes of a workout or five minutes of a race, increasing the rpm to flush the muscles, thus preventing the build up of lactic acid and having leaden legs at the beginning of the run split. Following a training time trial or a hard run, this can be done on a trainer or, for enhanced leg speed and bike handling skills, stationary rollers.

As a 10-year U.S. National Team member, Howard learned a valuable "anaerobic threshold" (AT) paceline training technique that all triathletes can use to get stronger while alone or on group rides. The lead rider goes out hard in the big ring at his AT, with the drafters behind him in their small rings. They rotate after a minute, with the new leader clicking into the big ring. Everyone gets a turn at the front. The key point here: Training in varying gears with a group helps to patch the holes in the cyclists' cardiovascular fitness. On top of that, it's a lot more fun than training alone, and teaches your muscles how to recover. The challenge of hanging on the wheel of a strong leader and trying to match his power when it's your turn as leader makes you much stronger quickly.

The same technique may also be used for active recovery between races or hard training sessions, says Howard. For example, one may do a short series of five to seven one-minute efforts in zone 3 to 4 while alternating between a small ring and a big one.

Feel the gear by putting the numbers on the back burner. A favorite routine on the same theme involves working on leg speed and power in the same workout to bolster the fast-twitch and slow-twitch responses simultaneously. The formulas may vary, but an example is hill repeats done on a 6 to 8 percent grade, with the length specific to the needs of the athlete. A typical workout might include two sets of the following:

1. a very low gear spin of 95 rpm
2. a big gear push, seated, of 30 rpm
3. race gear of 85 rpm

"I encourage my athletes to use one cog smaller gear than they think they need in both training and racing," says Howard. He promises you an easier, stronger ride, a seamless bike/run transition , and strong, un-wornout knees long past age 50.

"Plugging along in the big ring day after day in the aero position will eventually wreck your body and weaken the supporting muscles, thus making cycling a painful experience," he says, knowing personally of what he speaks. "I wish my coach had wired the frame-mounted shift lever down to keep me from abusing the big ring 30 years ago. I'm sure I would have more power and feel more comfortable now if he had taken such steps. In time, I have learned that raw power is a gift that must be savored and not wasted by pounding the big chain ring just because you can."

9

RUNNING TUTORIAL

HOW TO GET SAFE, INJURY-FREE FITNESS BY TRAIL RUNNING AND RAMPING UP SLOWLY

Between the years of 1989 and 1995, I participated in only one triathlon, but got pretty serious about running. I became decent at it, as running ability mirrors almost precisely what you put into it. Does being a good runner carry over into triathlon? Not exactly. I've known a few who made such a jump with virtual ease, but I was one of those who let the conceit of thinking my good running would automatically make me a good triathlete. It was most certainly a conceit. I entered a half Ironman triathlon with only run training in my body, and it was a long, long day. When I finally did get to the run leg, I was so exhausted by the swim and the bike I spent a lot of the run walking.

Actually, my favorite story of a pure runner getting tripped up by multisport is of a great friend of mine, Mike McManus. Mike was the best long-distance guy in the local circle of runners I knew in San Francisco back in the 1990s. He had a great work ethic and was extremely knowledgeable, two facts that forged his reputation as being competitive in distances as short as

1500 meters and as long as the marathon. But one weekend Mike decided to enter a duathlon of sorts, a race where you ran first and then swam. The first event was the run and, as anyone could have predicted, Mike established a huge lead. When he got to the point where he had to get into the frigid waters of the San Francisco Bay, he stood at the edge and hesitated, looking back over his shoulder. He finally got in and started swimming. Mike's swimming wasn't up to par with his running. When he tells the story, the image of the competitors raging past him like a school of sharks is pretty hilarious.

Oddly enough, Mike started biking a few years ago and has become a very good duathlete. He just needs to take on that swim to complete the trifecta.

If you've done some running or jogging in the past, that's great. If you haven't, rest assured that running is an activity in which you can make a lot of progress in a minimum of time. Because of the way you need to work against gravity, you can get an effective workout in as little as 30 minutes.

The most important principle to keep in mind about progressing with your run is to do it gradually. You need to find the sweet spot between consistency and patience. Your development as a runner requires that your muscles, tendons, and ligaments be exposed to small waves of increasing amounts of stress, so that in terms of strength and resilience they can keep several

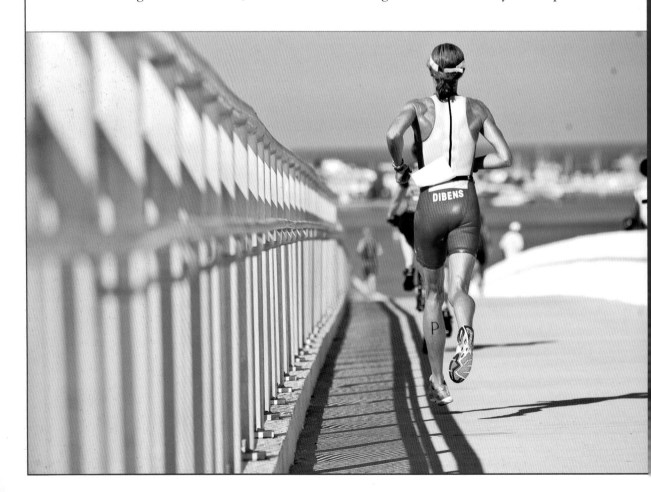

steps ahead of your training. Often, new runners get overexcited about the progress they can make quickly by running more, and wham, they get nailed with injuries like shin splints, Achilles tendon problems, and knee troubles.

Fortunately for you, triathlon helps prevent these pitfalls because active recovery is built-in, and with swimming and biking, you work muscle groups complementary to the muscles used in running. This is why, interestingly enough, more than a few injured, beat-up runners limp into the sport of triathlon, starved for some variety and cross-training.

If you have a weight problem, you'll should be encouraged about your choice of triathlon as the method of working off the pounds. When you're overweight, running alone puts a lot of stress on your joints that you might not be able to handle on day one. Triathlon training allows for a smoother, less injury-prone path to fitness by virtue of cross-training.

RUN FOR FUN: HIT THE TRAIL

Where to run is an important question for beginners. Treadmills can be boring, but you will know exactly how much distance you cover, at what pace, and as you improve over the weeks,

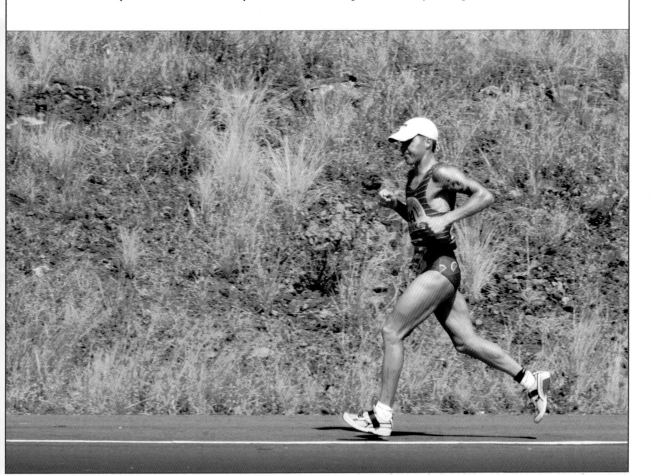

you'll see the numbers improve. Also, a treadmill has some give to it, so if you're worried about running on pavement, it's not a bad alternative at first. Eventually you'll want to work in some runs on the pavement to help adapt your body to the pounding because this is what you'll be facing in a race.

My favorite place to run is soft trails. You may want to avoid technical trails and hilly trails until you have a good year of experience, but once you feel confident, hit the dirt ASAP. Not only is the off-road running and triathlon scene exploding, but the benefits of trail running—both physical and mental—are too good to pass up. To tell you about the improved leg strength, reduction of injuries, and other great benefits of trail running, I defer to five-time Ironman finisher Luis Vargas, a MarkAllenOnline.com staff coach and a USAT Certified coach who loves doing it in the dirt.

More Strength, Fewer Injuries, Better Air

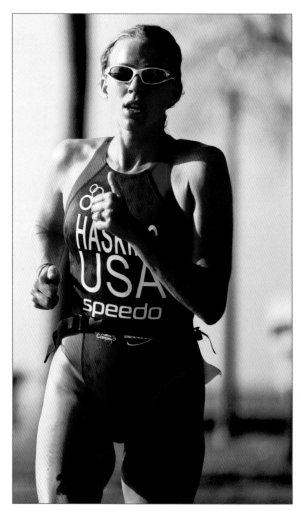

"Trail running will break your rhythm; it will slow you down but will build your strength in the process," says Vargas. "You may have to stop and turn, jump over a root or step up on to a rock." As triathletes, we have an advantage already as we have developed other leg muscles via cycling and swimming, but a bit of added leg strength is always welcomed.

Best of all, he says, the strength comes without any risk (if you don't count falling off a cliff, that is). Injuries are much less frequent than on pavement, for several reasons: while the softer surface reduces the pounding of pavement, the strengthening of more peripheral muscles by the uneven trail surfaces and lack of asphalt repetition typically reduces overuse injuries a great deal. "In fact," says Vargas, "many athletes who are frequently injured find that their aches and pains disappear when they add several days each week of trail running into their program." He warns that this is true only if you let your body adapt to trail running first. Introduce trail running gradually into your training.

Other benefits include improved ability to focus, better foot-eye coordination. ("If you don't concentrate you may find yourself on the ground," he says. "The good thing is that this ground is much softer.") Other benefits are obvious: No cars, and air you can't see. Your lungs will be much happier.

What to Bring: The Route, H$_2$0, and a Buddy

Trail running is great, but it still is out in the wild, reminds Vargas. To lessen the risks of being on the evening news, follow his off-road rules:

1. **Bike it:** Explore your trail on a mountain bike before you run it. Sometimes it can be fun to get lost in unknown territory, but you do not want your 40-minute run to turn into a two-hour ordeal. If you are directionally challenged, bring a fanny pack with a trail map, compass, and a cell phone. You can never be too safe.
2. **Slurp it:** Anytime you go into nature you should bring your own water or sports drink. You will need these fluids to replace all the fluids you lose. And if you choose to run in a very remote area, if you get lost or twist an ankle, the fluids may become life saving.

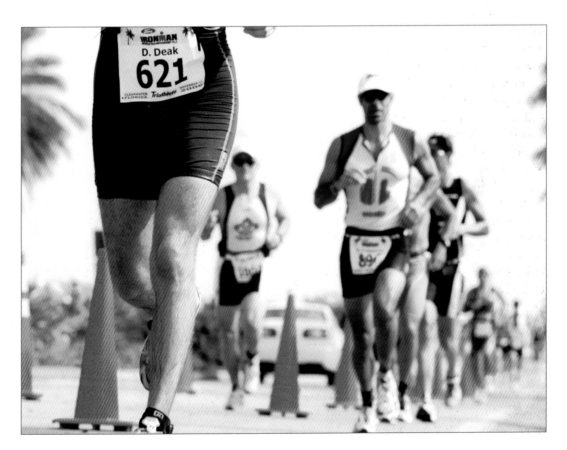

3. **Pal it:** Running with a buddy may not be critical if you run at your local city park where you can easily get help if needed; however, it is more important if you run in the wilderness. "I live in Colorado where bear, cougar, and moose encounters can happen," says Vargas. "Know your local wildlife and how to react if encountered. There is power in numbers."

Gear Up and Start Slow

You don't necessarily need to spring for trail running shoes. Some well-kept trails are so nicely maintained that your old street beaters will do. But as you get closer to ungroomed nature with uneven terrain, mud, sand, and water, specific trail running shoes offer more traction, stability and protection.

Your first trail runs can be exhilarating, but exhausting. Trail running is definitely more difficult than road running. Vargas's advice? "Slow down and gauge your effort with your heart rate monitor," he says. "Remember that minutes-per-mile on the road cannot be compared to trails."

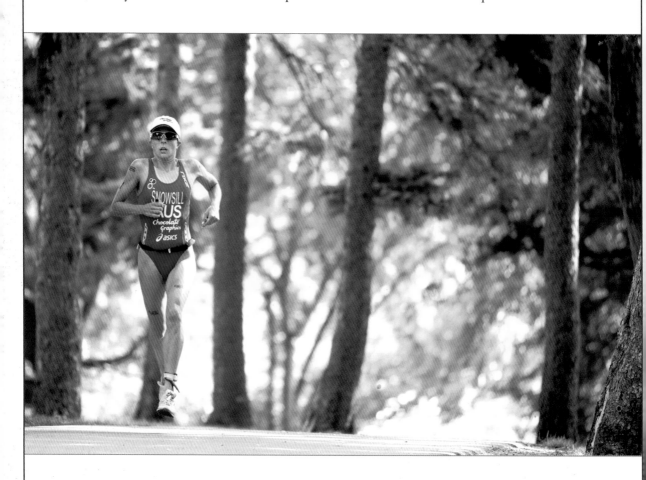

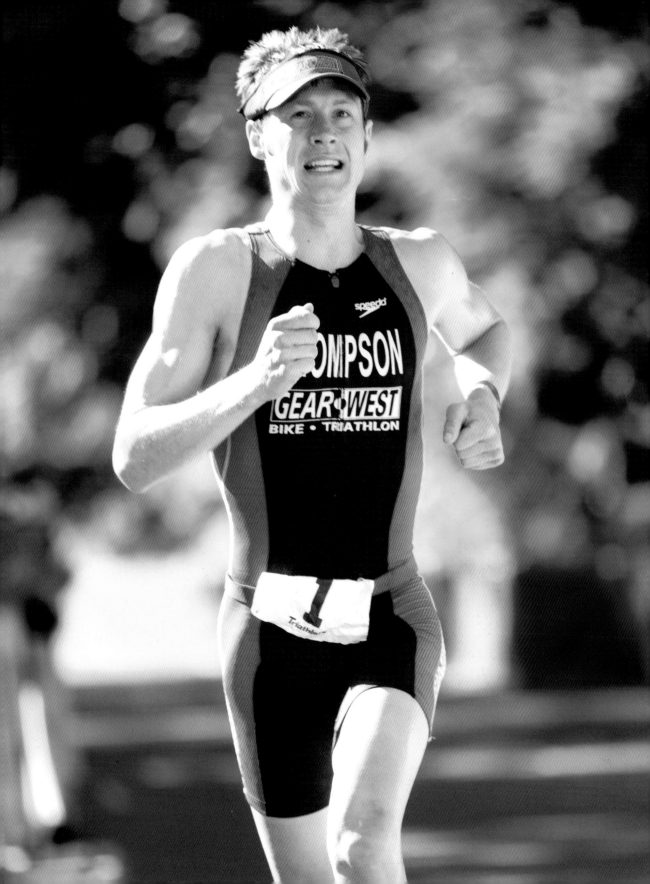

One of the biggest fears of trail running is twisted ankles and falls. Again, says Vargas, stay focused and shorten your stride when approaching any uneven or overly rocky areas. Stay light on your feet for better balance and recovery from slips on unstable surfaces. During the fall season watch for leaves that cover the ground and prevent you from seeing roots, rocks, and holes.

"Trail running can be that spice you need to revamp your running," says Vargas. "I can personally attest to its benefits. Whenever there is a snowstorm or a very rainy day I get out there. Not only do I have the entire trail to myself creating that one-with-nature feeling, but I also feel like I was getting a leg up on my competition by training on a day that they were most likely taking off."

Injury Prevention: Beating Shin Splints

Unfortunately, you can't talk about running without talking about injuries. Fortunately, the inherent cross-training involved in triathlon automatically reduces the frequency and severity of triathlete running-induced injuries compared to those of pure runners. But running is running, and injuries are still going to happen. One of the most common running injuries triathletes experience, especially when ramping up for big-mileage Ironman and half Ironman races, is shin splints.

Shin splints is a swelling and sharp pain on the inside part of the tibia (the shin bone) that tends to worsen during, but especially after, runs of rapidly increasing mileage. Pain that worsens after running and hurts when pressure is applied is the most common form of shin splints, called MTSS (medial tibial stress syndrome). According to Dr. Jordan D. Metzl, a sports medicine physician at the Hospital for Special Surgery in New York City and a 24-time marathon runner and three-time Ironman triathlete, those with low bone density and a pronating foot (meaning the foot rolls into the middle) are most vulnerable to this painful condition. Following are his recommendations for fixing the problem:

1. **Orthotics:** "It's not uncommon for one foot to pronate more than the other," says Metzl, "and this is usually the side where MTSS first appears." He believes that a good place to start correcting foot mechanics is through some off-the-shelf orthotics, found at many good running or triathlon stores (they can also go into bike shoes, where they make pedal strokes much more efficient).

2. **Back off, heal, then ramp up slowly:** Increasing mileage very quickly to try and catch up after falling behind is a sure-fire prescription for shin splints. "Most people can't tolerate more than a 5 to 10 percent increase in training volume per week," says Metzl. So if you start from a base of 10 miles a week, adding a mile a week is okay. Adding eight miles a week is not.

3. **Bone up:** Female athletes, beware: Thinning bones—due to genetics, low circulating estrogen levels from not menstruating for months at a time, and insufficient calcium intake (women need 1,300 to 1,500 milligrams of calcium per day, or four glasses of milk)—are a contributing factor to shin splints. Gals are more prone than males to

develop osteopenia (low bone density) and osteoporosis (very low bone density), which raise the risk of both swelling and more worrisome stress fractures. A thinning bone can withstand less stress before it starts to swell and, eventually, in more severe cases, can crack, producing a stress fracture. In the case of bone stress, the patient must stop running. "Pushing through the pain is a terrible idea," he says. "It can turn a stress injury into a stress fracture."

In a typical MTSS case, Metzl had a non-fractured shin splint patient stop running for a month, but continue cycling and swimming, which are both nonimpact activities. While her bone was healing, he tried to fix the causes of her injury with a pair of $25 orthotics for her running and biking shoes and instructed her to take calcium supplements to build strong bones. As her shin pain got better, she slowly began to run. By six weeks she was pain-free, and eight weeks later, she ran her race.

Dr. Metzl's Shin Splint To-Do list:

1. Prevent it by increasing mileage slowly. The golden rule is 10 percent per week.
2. Once injured, stop running and have the injury checked out.
3. Continue cross-training (swim and bike) if you can do so without pain.
4. Make sure your doctor figures out why this injury is happening. Is it your feet, your training, or your bone density? Make sure you find out before it happens again.
5. Listen to your body. Don't trust anyone but yourself to know when you are developing an injury.

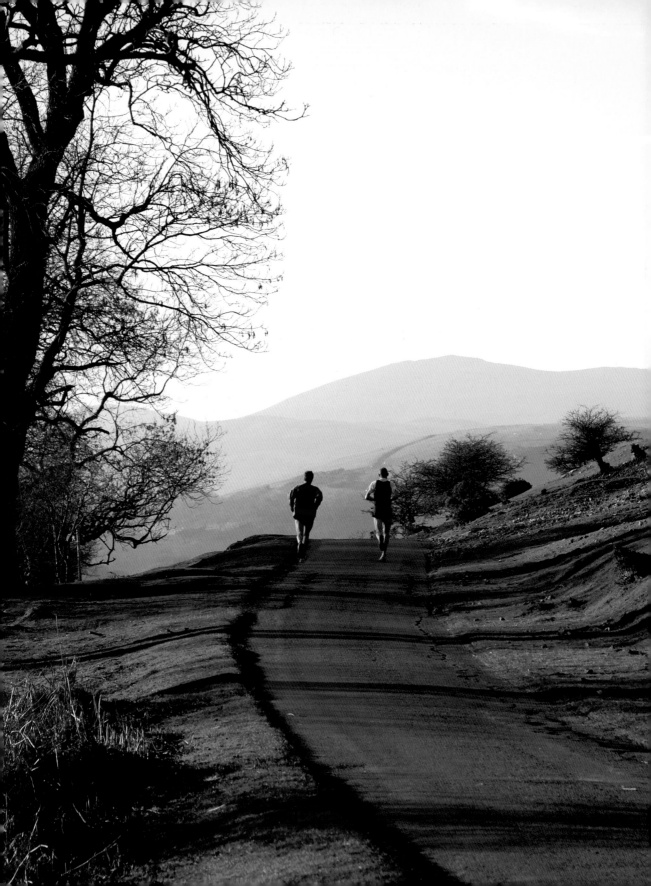

10

ADVANCED TRAINING FOR THE REST OF US

THE MUST-KNOW PRINCIPLES OF HEART RATE MONITORING, RECOVERY/OVERTAINING RULES, AND BASE TRAINING

It's a great time to be a newbie triathlete, because the doors of high-performance have been flung wide open. What used to be hidden, arcane knowledge available only behind the Iron Curtain or to elite Olympic and professional athletes is now out on Main Street, ready for the rest of us.

We're lucky: inexpensive technology and the wide dissemination of training principles has created a democratization of high performance. In other words, now you can be as good as you want to be. This chapter discusses three key performance concepts that are commonly referred to and used today by all triathletes and can make anyone's workouts more enjoyable and productive: heart rate monitoring, recovery/overtraining rules, and base training.

FIVE EASY STEPS TO HEART RATE MONITORING

If you're a beginner triathlete, heart rate monitoring will revolutionize the way you train—if you know how to interpret the numbers. Here's the quick and easy method to get it right from one of the true gurus of triathlon, marathoning, and heart rate training, Sally Edwards. In matters of the heart rate, few hold a candle to Edwards, who is a member of the Triathlon Hall of Fame, the national spokesperson for the Danskin Women's Triathlon, and the author of 12 books, including *The Heart Rate Monitor Guidebook* (1999). You can learn more about heart rate zone training by visiting her website, www.HeartZones.com.

Heart rate monitors (HRMs) are inexpensive and widely used today, but most people don't take full advantage of them, says Edwards. They see the data, but don't know how to interpret it. "If you don't know, it can't help you much," she says.

A few years ago, Edwards saw an example of this at a duathlon in Texas. She was approached by a triathlete who was curious as to why he couldn't sustain his heart rate on the second run, even though he had experienced no problems on the first run and bike legs. His HRM said it all: he was stressed on the second run. He'd gone too hard on the run and bike and had fatigued. Edwards told him that he was probably experiencing "cumulative fatigue" from the first two legs of the race and did the third one running on empty. He had burned through his stored energy and drained his muscles of power, speed, and strength.

The problem? "He didn't know how to process the information on his HRM to help diagnose his performance," says Edwards. "If he had known how to read it, he'd have known that

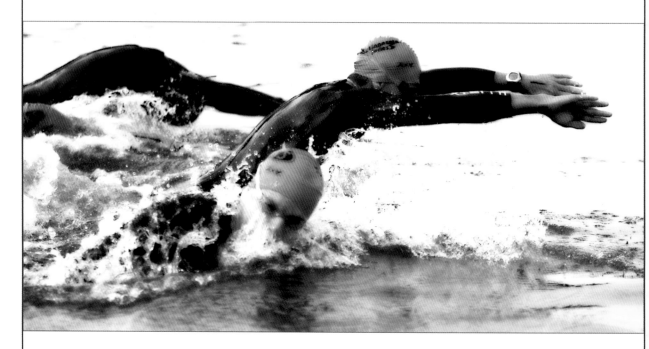

he went out too fast." Heart rate monitoring, she says, is more than just monitoring your heart beat; it's watching your heart in order to obtain analytical information.

Here's what Edwards says you need to know about how HRMs can help your with your triathlon workouts. She calls it the ABCs of heart rate training.

A: Answers

An HRM can tell you what percentage of your maximum heart rate you are currently training or racing at. It tells how much time you've spent in one of the five heart zones (see the chart below), plus how much fat, how many carbohydrates, and how many total calories you're burning. If you can understand the heart numbers on your monitor, it will answer your questions.

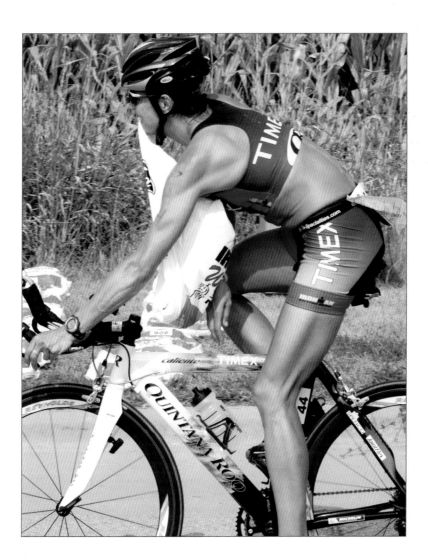

B: Benefits

For those who love to train "high and hard"—high intensity for long periods of time—an HRM can serve as a brake, slowing you down and keeping you optimized in your heart zones. If you like the "low and easy" type of training, an HRM is a powerful biofeedback device, telling you to increase your training intensity and add more physiological stress or increase the intensity. After all, that's what an HRM is measuring—relative physiological stress.

C: Control

Watching your HRM provides you with a control tool that accurately answers the question, "How hard am I training?"

Getting Started with Your HRM in Five Steps

1. **Find out your maximum heart rate.**

    Your heart rate maximum is the highest number of beats your heart can contract in one minute. Edwards, at age 52, after 30 years as a serious multisport athlete, had a max of 195 beats per minute running. Ned Overend, the XTERRA champion and three-time world mountain bike champion, has a maximum heart rate of 165 bpm; a 30 bpm difference. Lesson here? Maximum heart rate does not predict your success as a triathlete. It's just an anchor point used to set your heart zones.

    The most accurate way to find out your maximum heart rate is to go out hard and get a big number on your heart watch. If you don't want to experience that level of exercise stress, you can use a mathematical formula, which is not as accurate. Edwards' company, Heart Zones, has created a formula, which is the best one we've found yet:

    Maximum Heart Rate = your age in years, minus 5 percent of your body weight in pounds, plus 4 for men or 0 for women.

2. **Set your heart zones.**

    Once you have identified that number, set your heart zones, which are each 10 percent of your maximum heart rate. The Heart Zones chart offers an easy way to set your heart zones without having to do the math. Each of the heart zones is named after the benefit that you'll gain from getting your heart rate into that zone.

3. **Take a tour of your individual zones.**

    Strap on your heart rate monitor and start training. The first workouts I recommend are ones that allow you to "tour the zones." It's kind of like checking out a race course before doing an event; it helps you know what to expect. Next, do your favorite workout and see what zones you have been training in. Finally, try a new workout on an indoor bike or a treadmill and see which of the five heart zones you are training in.

4. **Plug your heart rate zones into your training schedule.**

    With your heart rate zones now in place, you can more accurately conquer the specifics of a workout goal. If the purpose of the workout is to develop your aerobic base, you can set the upper and lower limits of your monitor's alarms to the corresponding numbers of your zone 3 parameters. And if the objective of a workout is to spend twenty minutes in your anaerobic zone (zone 4) you now have a more exact way to develop your ability to exercise at the higher intensities that preparation for racing demands. Ideally, you're in a situation where you're working with a coach whose approach is grounded in the language of exercise physiology. But even if you're self-coached, most of the better triathlon training books available today organize triathlon training programs with heart rate zones in mind.

5. **Plot your heart rate information from your workout in your logbook.**

    The value of your logbook takes on a new depth with the addition of monitoring your heart rate during training. Imagine being able to look at the speeds that you put forth in certain workouts of a past training year with what you're doing at similar times during this training year. Plotting the numerics of your training sessions throughout the training cycles of the year is a great way to spot which types of approaches are working for you and which are working against you. This process also helps you and your coach to develop pinpoint methods of tapering for important races.

    Once you've started watching your heart rates and monitoring your workouts, you'll probably discover the answers to your most vexing fitness questions. If you've been killing yourself trying to lose those last five to 10 pounds of body fat, you might find that you're simply working in too high of a zone.

    Or, if you're like Michael, and can't get your heart rate to the number you want in a race, you need to spend more time training at your racing heart rate number so you can sustain it during a race. Fading at the end of a race usually means that you haven't built on top of your aerobic foundation, a layer of zone 4 threshold training. Using a monitor strengthens the body, prevents premature old age, and prolongs the energy of youth.

Heart Zone Training Chart

Heart Rate Zones

Zone Number	% of Maximum Heart Rate	
1	50%–60%	Fat-burning zone
2	60%–70%	Recovery zone
3	70%–80%	Aerobic zone
4	80%–90%	Anaerobic zone
5	90%–100%	Red Line Zone

Example: If your max heart rate is 190, your zones would read as the following:

Zone 1: HR 95–114 beats per minute
Zone 2: HR 115–133
Zone 3: HR 134–152
Zone 4: HR 153–171
Zone 5: HR 172–Max (This zone is best left to extremely fit athletes. Triathletes in general, Ironman elites included, have little reason to train in this zone.)

WHY RECOVERY IS KEY

"Recovery is when your body actually grows stronger and more efficient. It is when the benefits of your hard training are realized," says Bob Kersee, track and field coach of 24 Olympic medal–winning performances. "Working hard is easy, everyone knows how to work hard, but those who know how to recover hard (well) are the ones who win."

Robert Forster, a physical therapist who operates the Phase IV high-performance training center in Santa Monica, California (www.phase-iv.net), knows Bob Kersee well. From the early 1980s, they worked together preparing some of the world's best athletes, including Florence Griffith Joyner and Jackie Joyner-Kersee. His exposure to training methods of top Olympians from former Eastern Bloc nations, combined with his physical therapy expertise, led him to a deep appreciation of the science of Periodization Training, a systematic way of developing fitness in a scientifically rational, stair-step-like progressive sequence. A key to that sequence is the most important aspect of training, without which all your hard work is futile: recovery. Recovery is what triathletes don't do well: take an off-day.

Why is an off-day—or even an easy week—important? "Following periods of hard work, fatigue and an initial decrease in performance occur before the body adapts and emerges stronger and more efficient," says Forster. "However, this occurs only if time for recovery is provided." In other words, don't rest and you'll pay the price with fatigue, mental and physical burnout, and less-than-peak performance when it counts.

The concept is not hard to understand. In Periodization, you "overload"—build up bigger and bigger training miles over three weeks, then follow that with a week of decreased workload, or recovery.

Recovery is of particularly great value to beginners. That's because their structural system (tendons, bone, fascia) is not well-developed from years of training. Getting in the recovery time is essential to strengthening that structure.

So even though you may be super-enthusiastic about getting into the triathlon lifestyle, you can't go hog wild. Don't look at an off-day as laziness. Timed correctly, it helps make you stronger. Don't do it and you'll run the risk of contracting the disease rampant in the triathlon world: overtraining.

HOW TO PREVENT OVERTRAINING

1. **Put rest on the schedule:**
   Nip overtraining in the bud with built-in rest and recovery periods at regular intervals in your training program. Don't trust your yourself to know when you need rest; program it in. The likelihood of becoming overtrained increases when un-coached, over-enthused athletes increase their training load after perceiving a plateau or decrease in performance.

2. **Slow and steady build up during Base Training:**
   As you build your base in a slow and deliberate manner with low-intensity exercise, you are literally building the structures that allow it to handle more rigorous aerobic training

down the road. In addition to upgrading your bones and connective tissue, vascularization (more capillaries) arises to transport blood, oxygen, and nutrients to growing muscles and to send waste products away. The prolonged low-intensity exercise also improves the athlete's ability to produce energy aerobically by burning fat, which it has a huge supply of, rather than the less numerous carbs, which are better saved for later. Train yourself to burn more fat, and you delay or avoid glycogen depletion, also known as bonking.

Where does recovery enter the Base Training equation? Simply this: As you slowly strengthen your body, you will be giving yourself insurance. That insurance manifests itself as fewer injuries in the future and decreased recovery time when the exercise intensity increases later in the season as you peak for races. And when the race is over, you'll recover faster. And that translates to harder training and better performances later while staving off the dreadful overtrained state.

3. **Constantly vary your workouts:**
The human body is an amazingly adaptive machine. Put stress on it, and it gets stronger. Ironically, however, it gets stronger only for a limited period of time if it is confronted with certain types of stress (in your case, exercise). Fact: after about six to eight weeks of a certain type of exercise, full adaptation occurs. So to stimulate further growth, you have to alter the exercise. This keeps the body constantly off balance and forces further adaptation while avoiding staleness. Conveniently, this variety in training also avoids mental burnout and keeps focus and motivation high. Volume and intensity variation characteristic to each phase of Periodization Training creates a constantly evolving program, which keeps the body and mind fresh.

4. **Active Recovery and Stretching:**
I hope I didn't give you the wrong idea. Recovery doesn't mean turning back into a couch potato for a week. One day off might be the most total off-time called for. Most of recovery is "active," involving less volume and intensity of exercise. "Light adaptation workouts stimulate recovery better than rest alone," says Forster. "Light workouts are akin to the self-cleaning oven where the heat is turned up but no roast is placed inside. Light workouts provide the body the same opportunity to do house cleaning functions without having to recover from the damaging effects of a new workout."

Stretching sessions before and particularly after light recovery workouts are more productive when unencumbered by the tightness that would otherwise occur following hard workouts. In this way your stretching efforts go further toward elongating connective tissue and helping tendons and ligaments heal and grow stronger. A good indication of when your structural system is recovered and ready for another hard workout is when the stiffness from the last hard workout is absent.

5. **Self-massage:**
Have you ever heard anyone say that he or she didn't like a good massage? Your athletic, triathlon-training body loves massage for a reason: It aids recovery after workouts.

Manipulation of the muscles and tissues increases blood flow, breaks adhesions, and promotes adaptation of connective tissue.

"No specific knowledge or training is necessary," says Forster. "Just take some lotion and begin rubbing your calf and thigh muscles, front and back. You will feel the fatigue and tension leave your body." When coupled with stretching and icing sore areas, these self-recovery techniques can make a very significant contribution to the adaptive process you seek, i.e., increased fitness.

Commandments of Recovery and Prevention of Overtraining

1. **Build Adequate Base**—early season training builds infrastructure that supports hard work and recovery efforts later in the season.
2. **Built-In Rest Periods**—your training program must have built in recovery weeks following every two to three weeks of harder exercise. This includes the Base Training Phase. Also, always allow for a period of detraining at the end of your competitive season to allow all systems to recover.
3. **Vary Intensity and Volume**—every eight weeks, change the nature of your workouts to keep the body off balance and force further adaptation. Remember, volume must decrease as intensity increases.
4. **Stretch Before and After Every Workout**—stretching prepares the body for exercise and minimizes the damage created during workouts. Stretching after workouts wrings the waste products out of the muscles and returns muscles to their normal resting length, therefore avoiding maladaptive muscle and tendon shortening.
5. **Self-massage Before and After Workouts**—with this simple technique you can prevent damage and promote recovery like the pros.
6. **Ice Sore and Tight Areas**—ice reduces inflammation, muscle tightness and spasm, and allows muscles to relax and recover better. Ice helps avoid injuries and treats minor irritations before they develop into overuse syndromes.
7. **Keep Muscle Glycogen Topped Off**—carbohydrate stores in the muscle and liver (glycogen) become the limiting factor in endurance events lasting greater than 90 minutes. Maintain adequate levels with sport drink supplementation during exercise and begin replenishing within 15 minutes after workouts. Back-to-back long or difficult workouts can create a constant glycogen depleted state.

TECHNIQUE-FOCUSED BASE TRAINING

For basic training and advanced training, no one explains it better than Matt Fitzgerald, a coach, longtime *Triathlete Magazine* editor, and a contributor to *Runner's World, Men's Health*, and other national magazines. My longtime coeditor has examined training in every which way. I think he's a genius—and I might say that even if I didn't know that he'd be reading this. In this compelling study, Matt examines the eternal question, What is the best measure of true triathlon fitness?

Conventional wisdom holds that the foundation of triathlon performance is basic cardio-vascular fitness—the aerobic capacity needed to swim, bike, and run for sustained durations at a moderate intensity.

But Fitzgerald makes the case that the best aerobic capacity in the world is useless without good technique. Not just decent technique, but truly good technique that can take advantage of that hard-won aerobic fitness.

So his angle is simple: The base phase of triathlon training should begin with a technique focus period—several weeks of training that are focused above all else on cultivating better swim, bike, and run technique. He says that technique and aerobic don't mix well; that there's no time later in the year to focus on technique, anyway; and that proper technique is great insurance against injuries.

Ultimately, Fitzgerald thinks that convention aerobic base training should not begin at the beginning of the training cycle but immediately following four to six weeks of a very different type of training designed to improve technique. The bottom line: you need to swim, bike, and run *right* before you try to swim, bike, and run *a lot*. So, how is this done?

The Technique Focus Training Plan

There are three types of training you should do during a technique focus period: conscious control workouts, drills, and functional strength training.

Conscious Control

In technique sports such as golf and tennis, participants are accustomed to improving their technique by repetitively practicing specific movement patterns copied from the best players. You can and should improve your swim, bike, and run technique in the same way.

The first step is to identify a specific flaw in your technique or, put another way, to identify an aspect of correct technique that is missing from your own. This may require the assistance of a coach or other observer. One example of a common and correctable technique flaw is pronounced heel striking in running.

Step two is to begin playing around with incorporating this technique modification into your swim stroke, pedal stroke, or running stride. Our example of pronounced heel strik-ing results from allowing the feet to land too far ahead of the body. If you have this flaw, you'll want to practice retracting your leg (drawing it backward) in the moments before the foot lands, so that it lands more underneath your body and consequently more towards the midfoot.

Once you've gotten a basic feel for the new technique, your task is to repeat this improved movement pattern as exactly as possible with every single stroke or stride until it has become automatic, which will probably take several weeks.

This process requires great concentration and focus. Therefore, I recommend that you work on just one technique modification at a time in each discipline. It's also important to swim, bike, and run for only short periods of time when using conscious control to groove a technique change. If you go too long, fatigue (which will come more quickly than usual, as you're using some muscles in new ways) and/or inattention will cause you to revert back to old habits.

If you're worried about maintaining basic cardiovascular fitness during the technique focus period, resist the temptation to swim, bike, or run more and instead do some form of cross-training, such as using an elliptical trainer.

Drills

The difference between conscious control and drills is that, in the former, you swim, ride, or run normally while consciously controlling one specific component of the movement; whereas in the latter, you break down the normal swim stroke, pedal stroke, or stride into basic components and work on developing proper technique in each, one at a time.

Drills are, of course, common in swimming. In a typical swim workout, a short drill set is sandwiched between the warm-up and the main set. During your technique focus period, the drill set should become your main set. Increase the variety and volume of drills you do and scrap the intervals altogether.

It's important that you also do cycling and running drills during your technique focus period. Here are some suggestions:

Running Drills

High Knees

Run with a fast cadence and highly exaggerated knee lift, bringing your thighs up parallel to the ground with each stride. Continue for 30 seconds.

Butt Kicks

Run in place or slowly forward while keeping your thighs perpendicular to the ground, trying to kick yourself in the butt with your heels. Continue for 30 seconds.

Leap Running

Run with the longest, leaping strides you can achieve (like the first two jumps in a track and field triple jump). Continue for 30 seconds.

Cycling Drills

Single-Leg Pedaling

On a wind trainer or a stationary bike, pedal in a low gear (low resistance level) with a single leg while keeping your other leg out of the way (e.g., on a chair). Go for one minute and then switch legs. Repeat the drill a few times more.

Sample Technique Focus Period Schedule

Monday	Tuesday	Wednesday	Thursday	Friday	Saturday	Sunday
Off	Swim 400y CC W/U 800y Drills 400y CC C/D	Bike 0:30 Spin Scan or Power Cranks 0:10 drills	Run 0:10 CC W/U 0:10 Drills 0:10 CC C/D	Swim 400y CC W/U 800y Drills 400y CC C/D	Bike 1:00 CC Ride	Run 0:10 CC W/U 0:10 Drills 0:10 CC C/D
	Functional Strength		Functional Strength		Functional Strength	

Key
CC = Conscious control
W/U = Warm-up
C/D = Cool-down

Spinning Out

Gradually increase your pedaling cadence over the course of several minutes, in a very low gear, until you reach maximum rpm, which you then maintain for 30 to 60 seconds. Try to keep your butt from bouncing in the saddle.

In addition to drills, there are special tools you can use to improve your pedal stroke. Two that I recommend for use during the technique focus period are CompuTrainer's SpinScan (www.CompuTrainer.com), which allows you to watch a real time, graphic representation of your pedal stroke during an indoor ride; and PowerCranks (www.PowerCranks.com), a special type of pedal crank that forces you to pedal with a perfectly symmetrical stroke.

Functional Strength Training

Various muscular imbalances also contribute to technique flaws and the overuse injuries that result from them. For example, weak hip abductors can cause the pelvis to tilt laterally on impact during running, placing stress on the hips and knees. All the drills and conscious control in the world won't allow you to swim, bike, and run correctly if you don't have the right musculature to support good form.

Functional strength training can give you the muscle balance and joint stability you need to improve your technique. A strength exercise is considered functional if it approximates a movement pattern that is used in swimming, cycling, or running. Such specificity allows it to have functional carryover to that discipline. An example is walking lunges, which mimic both gait and pedal stroke patterns.

A little strength training can go a long way for triathletes, but a technique focus period is the best time to do the greatest amount of strength training. I recommend three sessions per week lasting 30 to 40 minutes apiece, as in the sample schedule on page 105. Later, I'll provide a complete functional strength workout to do during your technique focus period the next month.

11

12 WEEKS TO YOUR FIRST RACE

A FOOLPROOF THREE-MONTH PLAN TO TAKE YOU FROM BEGINNER ATHLETE TO FIRST-TIME SPRINT TRIATHLETE

Anyone who thinks they're too old, too weak, too fat, or too lazy to become a triathlete is vastly misinformed. Every year the ranks of triathlon swell in number as a fresh generation of triathletes migrates into the sport, motivated by all reasons imaginable. What do they discover? That training for a triathlon is not as hard as it's often made out to be; by mixing a little planning with the desire to get fit and participate will often breed a streak of discipline that shines like a ray of sunlight at daybreak.

This plan is designed for the sheer beginner. To get started, pack your bags for the journey by clicking off the following basic steps:

Step 1: **Get your doctor's okay.** Most places, even a 17-year-old has to get a doctor's permission to try out for a sport. Even one as physically mild as golf. Get a physical, and tell your doctor about this triathlon thing you're up to (ideally your doctor is a runner or triathlete—someone who gets it). Use this training program as a springboard to a clean bill of health, as well as your new venture into multisport.

Step 2: **Find a training partner if possible.** Even if you and a compatible training partner can only hook up on weekends, a training partner makes a phenomenal difference in getting your butt out the door. And as triathletes around the world have commonly discovered, training with friends is the best part about being in the sport.

Step 3: **Commit to a full year of being a triathlete.** This program is a 12-week kickoff into triathlon life, but if your goal is to transform your habits for good, it's important to declare at the start that you and your partner will train for a full year. According to sports psychologist Dr. Denis Waitley, following a new discipline for a year is the best way of turning it into a lifelong habit.

Step 4: **Find a target race at least three months out.** The program mentioned here is meant to prepare your body to finish a standard sprint distance triathlon, like the Danskin Series races: a quarter-mile swim, 12-mile bike, and five-kilometer run. Sprint triathlons are often

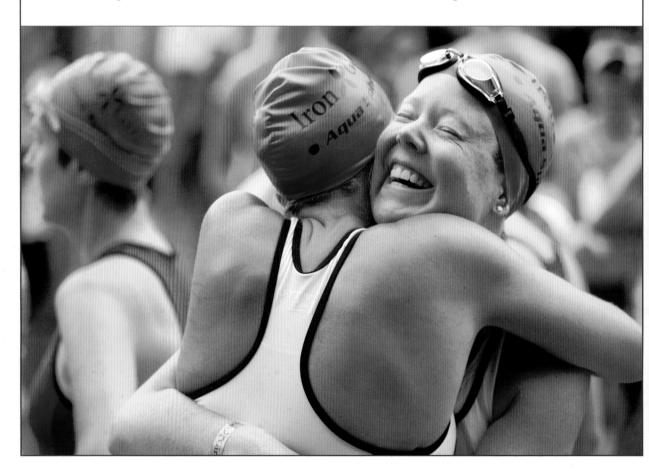

a part of the weekend schedules of major triathlon festivals around the country. You can find them through various race calendar websites, like www.Active.com, or by using *Triathlete Magazine*'s North American Event Guide.

Step 5: **Set up your logbook and first workout.** If you performed the Basic Training program in this book, continue to use the logbook you started there.

Step 6: **The Basic Training program should have put you in a condition where this following program is a natural progression.** If you feel like you need more time, take it, and continue to follow the last few weeks of the Basic Training program until your confidence is high.

SIX KEYS TO TRAINING

1. **Slowly build the base:** Perform your workouts at an easy pace. If you can't comfortably maintain a conversation while running or biking, you're going too hard. After you graduate from your first triathlon, the time will be ripe for introducing small amounts of

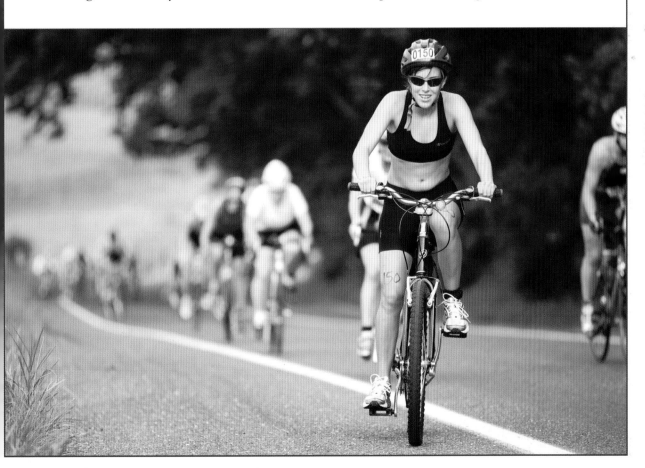

intensity to your training. But the bedrock of any good triathlon program is composed primarily of low-intensity cardiovascular work—popularly known as base training. A fast finishing sprint in a triathlon is worthless unless you have the aerobic base to get you into the position to outsprint a competitor. Base is where it's at.

2. **Chill-out on Mondays:** That's your rest day. Take this day off.

3. **Stay cool in the pool:** When swimming, don't worry about speed. The key is working on good technique and staying relaxed in the water. The most important thing is to get in the pool every week.

4. **No wimpy weekends:** The key workouts of this program are on the weekend. By adding a few minutes to the previous weekend's bike and run, your body slowly adapts to the stress by increasing cardiovascular efficiency (including the body's ability to burn fat) and musculoskeletal strength. This is what it's all about.

5. **Observe the taper:** During the last week of the program, training times drop as you taper for your race. If your race is more than 12 weeks away, simply repeat weeks 10

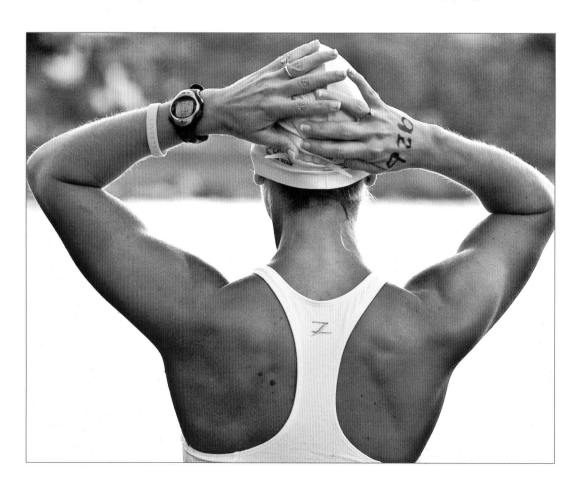

and 11 until you're one week out from the big day. Then follow the taper, eat plenty of healthy food, and get plenty of rest. On race day, have fun as you cross the finish line into the world of triathlon.

6. **Stick to the plan:** The workout schedule laid out in the chart below is a logical, proven formula that will get you in race shape—but only if you do it. The chart is separated into two six-week chunks. Each workout is listed in minutes. Remember: This isn't about setting records; it is about putting in enough raw time to be able to complete a short-distance triathlon.

Where to go from here? After you finish your first race, take a couple of well-deserved days off and then get right back into it. Immediately set another race goal. If you like the sprint distance, stick to this basic schedule and ramp up the speed to continue challenging yourself. If you have the desire to push it up to Olympic distance, check out Coach D's hardcore 12-week program in chapter 15.

Whatever challenges you choose, make training consistently your mantra. Consider hooking up with a local triathlon club. Get a subscription to *Triathlete Magazine*. You've got the fitness and the finisher's medal to prove it, and the feeling's too good to give up. You're an honest-to-goodness triathlete now!

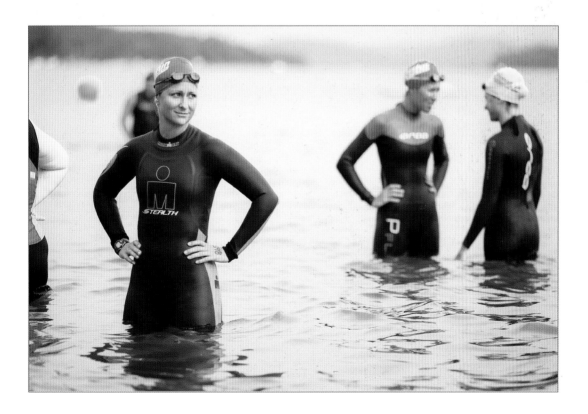

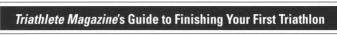
Twelve Weeks To Completing Your First Sprint Triathlon

	1	2	3	4	5	6
First Six Weeks						
Saturday: Run	15	20	25	30	35	40
Sunday: Bike	30	40	45	50	55	60
Tuesday: Swim	15	15	20	20	25	25
Wednesday: Run	15	15	20	20	25	25
Thursday: Bike	20	20	25	30	30	35
Friday: Swim	15	15	20	20	20	25
Second Six Weeks						
Saturday: Run	35	45	50	55	60	40
Sunday: Bike	45	65	70	75	80	80
Tuesday: Swim	25	30	30	35	40	20
Wednesday: Run	25	30	30	35	35	15
Thursday: Bike	30	35	40	30	40	20
Friday: Swim	15–30	15–30	15–30	15–30	15–30	OFF: Tomorrow race day*

*If Sunday is your race day, go for a 15-minute jog on Friday and take Saturday off.

12
RACE DAY

THE JITTER-FREE GUIDE TO YOUR FIRST OFFICIAL DAY AS A TRIATHLETE

It's here. Maybe it's been eighteen weeks in the making. Maybe 18 years. The big day. Race day.

This chapter addresses the most pressing, anxiety-ridden aspects of race day. It will tell you how to warm up for the swim. It'll tell you what, when, and how to eat on this day—including a detailed analysis of how to handle the all-important bike leg. And so you can dream of bigger things to come, it lays out pre-race recommendations for the Big Show, the Hawaii Ironman, which can be applied to any Ironman-distance race.

But before we get into all that, a word to the wise: don't screw it up before you leave the house. Four days beforehand, start checking off your laundry list, starting with peripherals and in order of the events. Put everything in one corner of your house that you know the dog won't disturb.

THE RACE DAY LAUNDRY LIST

Accessories
Sunglasses
Sunscreen
Sports lubricant
Energy bars
GU energy gel
Waterbottles filled with electrolyte replacement
Towel
Racebelt

The Swim

Wetsuit
Swimsuit
Goggles

The Bike

Bicycle (tuned up, of course)
Helmet
Gloves
Bike shoes
Bike shorts
Seat bag with repair tools

The Run

Running shoes
Visor

Make sure you know the route to the race. Set your alarm for the middle of the night. Arrive at the race venue two hours early.

THE FOURTH EVENT: RACE DAY NUTRITION

Your bike is tuned up. Your running shoes are outfitted with lacelocks. Your new wetsuit fits perfectly. Your training is flawless. But whatever you do, don't forget the fourth event: eating. In-race nutrition can be the difference between a triumph and a disaster.

For long and ultradistance triathlons, proper nutrition during a race can make or break an effort. The Hawaii Ironman offers a supreme example of this. The field of 1,800 athletes is packed with exceptionally talented, driven, and hard-working triathletes from around the world. They arrive for the race at the peak of their game. Yet every year, due to the duration, intensity, heat, and wind of the Hawaii Ironman, on race day competitors run into trouble, sometimes being forced to drop out, because of mistakes related to nutrition.

Of course, the Hawaii Ironman takes athletes anywhere up to 17 hours to finish (seventeen hours is the offical cut off). This is a lot of time to be exercising in a place known for heat, humidity, and harsh winds. Drink or eat too much or too little, too fast or not the right thing, and stomachs go into rebellion. Perhaps the most common ailment at Ironman-distance events is hyponatremia, a condition in which sodium balance is out of whack because an athlete has not been taking in enough salt.

For every triathlete aspiring to race triathlons of half Ironman distance or longer, nutrition technique should be a major part of his or her race preparations. However, fortunately for those out to complete their first sprint-distance triathlon, you will not need to worry as much about this. Because you'll be exercising for a more manageable amount of time, race nutrition won't be fraught with as many hazards. However, it will still require your attention. Let's look at several common sprint distance tris and what they entail.

Tri-for-Fun: Pleasanton, California. 400-yard swim, 11-mile bike, 3.1-mile run.
Danskin Triathlon Denver: Denver, Colorado. 1/2-mile swim, 12-mile bike, 3.1-mile run.
Timberman Short Course Tri: Lake Winnipesaukee, New Hampshire. 1/3-mile swim, 15-mile bike, 3-mile run.

These races typify the general range of sprint-distance triathlons, and are what the 12-week training program in this book prepares you for. Beginning triathletes can expect to finish anywhere between one and a half hours to three hours, depending on the exact distance and, of course, current state of fitness and ability. It's your first tri, so it's all about finishing with a smile on your face.

To have that smile on your face, you will need to carry out five basic missions when it comes to nutrition. If you do these, you should be okay.

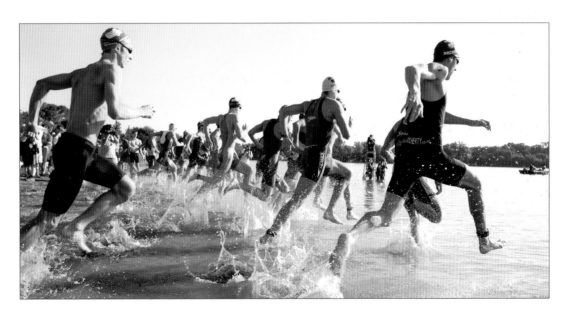

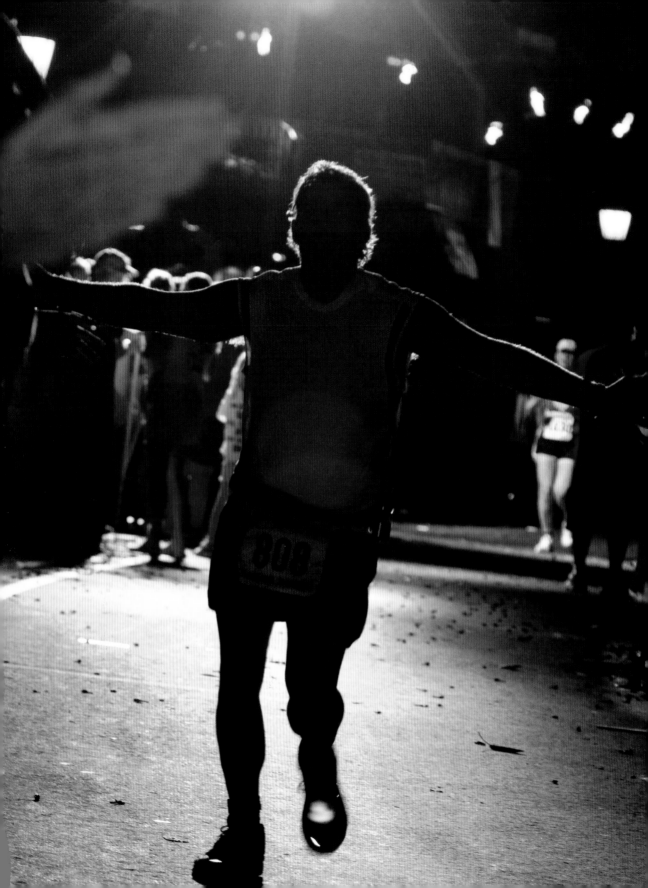

1. **Eat a proper diet during the week of the race:**
   Be certain to drink plenty of water during the week to maximize your hydration. Plenty of fruit and vegetables; complex, whole grain carbohydrates; and lean proteins; but don't overeat during the week, because you will be tapering. One of the most common mistakes is missing meals in the two days before the race because of traveling, hotels, and the challenge of finding groceries or proper restaurants in an unfamiliar place. If you're driving a long way, pack up a large cooler with good food and drinks to make sure you have a backup plan right by your side.

2. **Carb-up:**
   Eat a carbohydrate-rich meal—something you eat frequently and know your stomach will be in agreement with—in the late afternoon or early in the evening on the day before your race. Pasta is the famous pre-race dinner, and it's always a safe choice. Avoid eating this meal late in the evening and do not overeat. You want to give it plenty of time to clear your digestive system so that it may be used as energy during race day (as opposed to forcing frequent bathroom stops during the race).

3. **Do breakfast:**
   About two hours before your race, eat an easy to digest pre-race breakfast. A bowl of cereal or oatmeal is a good choice, topped off with a sports bar. Make sure this meal is high in carbs.

4. **Sports drink in-race:**
   During the race, you drink a large bottle of sports drink during the bike ride. Taking sips every 15 minutes or so will help stave off dehydration and replace some of the energy

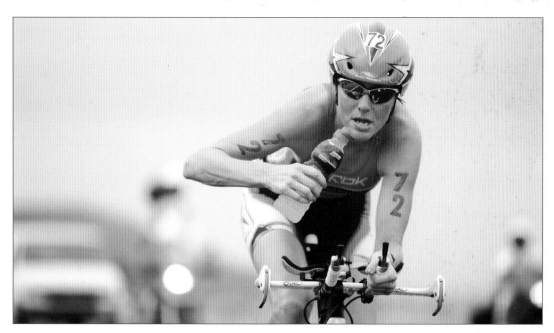

you're burning. The hotter and more humid the conditions are, the more you should pay attention to drinking.

5. **Walk this way:**

During the run, walk through each aid station and drink sports drink and water, and feel free to snack on energy bars and fruit. The golden rule of racing triathlons is this: Do what you need to do to stay comfortable. Food, drink, sunscreen, and Vaseline are popular items at aid stations. If you feel sick, dizzy, or have any other sort of uncomfortable symptom, ask volunteers at the aid station if there's a physician or nurse who could check you out.

After the race, continue eating and drinking to enhance recovery, and reward yourself with a nutritious lunch and dinner that day.

These are fairly common suggestions in the world of triathlon for the beginning triathlete entering a short distance tri. If you know you have a touchy stomach, or are particularly worried about getting this right, sports nutritionists and dieticians are incredible resources to help you dial in your individual idiosyncrasies.

THE 15 MUST-DOS OF RACE DAY EATING

Adhering to solid principles of sports nutrition science won't make you faster on race day, but it will help you not slow down. In addition to a review of the basics of what you should do on and around race day, included below is an overview the ever-expanding choice of bars, gels, and drinks on the market that are made with the triathlete in mind.

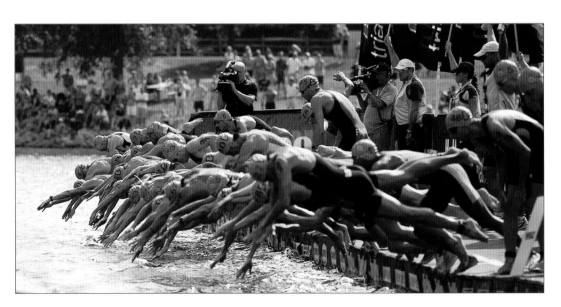

1. **Prepare your fuel-intake logistics in accordance with your race distance.** If you're racing a sprint distance triathlon and don't expect to be on the course more than an hour, you'll be wasting your time chewing up three sports bars on the bike ride. Outside of a light breakfast, water and sports drinks will provide more than enough energy and hydration. But the longer the event, the more critical race day nutrition becomes. Half Ironmans and Ironmans require preparing for the run by taking in calories, fluids, and sodium during the bike. This is best done by metronome-like grazing every 15 to 30 minutes, aiming for about 300 calories per hour for an Ironman and 150 calories per hour in an Olympic-distance event. We highly recommend talking to a registered dietician or sports nutritionist to analyze your weight against the needs of your race distances and determine precise numbers.

2. **For longer races, practice eating and drinking during training.** Success in long triathlons is dictated by your ability to stay in a positive physical state through as much of the race as possible. In other words, keep yourself feeling good. In this concern, nutrition is the key to the Kryptonite lock. In preparing for an event, do as astronauts do: simulate. Using workouts as "practice races," consume your target number of ounces and calories while on long bike rides and runs. Get in the habit of following a strict schedule to build discipline for the race. This sort of specific work may help those who are plagued with hurling troubles to teach your stomach how to keep things down until it's converted into blood sugar.

3. **Drink early in the race, whether you're thirsty or not.** Your sense of thirst cannot be trusted as a means of staying hydrated. The first thing to keep in mind is to go out of

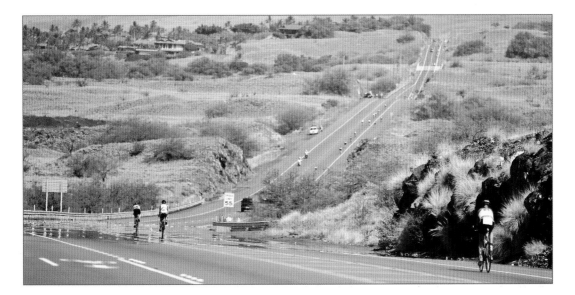

your way to drink fluids every 15 minutes during the bike, even though you don't feel a hint of thirst. Waiting for the onset of thirst means that you're allowing yourself to fall into a hole, which means performance weakens and you'll be faced with the task of digging yourself out.

4. **Find out what's going to be on the race course and do work to replicate it in training.** Save the potential sense of surprise for an upcoming birthday. Find out what drinks and eats are going to be provided on the course, and work them into your rotation during training.

5. **Become your own scientist.** Individual sweat rates, race conditions, and exercise intensity cloud the possibility of saying "you should drink exactly so many ounces of fluid per hour." On average, a triathlete should shoot for 500 mililiters per hour, and the perfect fluid is a sports drink with a 6 to 8 percent carbohydrate concentration that is relatively high in sodium. Again, working with a nutrition specialist is a worthwile investment for guiding you in maximing results from this process.

6. **Properly time your last carbo-loading meal.** This principle addresses the question, *How can I minimalize my time spent in Porta Potties during the race?* The answer is part science and part individual variation, the goal being to satisfactorily stuff your deeper energy reserves to the hilt without starting the race with an overload of material still working it's way through the conveyor belt of digestion. One way to do this is to confine your diet to carbohydrates that digest quickly and easily. Rice, potatoes, pasta, cookies, and white bread are the ticket. The more refined, believe it or not, the better. Post your final large carbohydrate meal approximately 18 hours before the start of the race, and thereafter restrict yourself to smaller rounds of food.

7. **Be prepared on the road.** When traveling to an out-of-town event, bring an assortment of healthy foods with you to avoid being forced to eat fastfood or junk food. If you're eating your meals at a gas station, you know you're in trouble.

8. **Experiment with stronger solutions of race drinks to prepare for aid stations.** In other words, be ready for anything. There's no guarantee that the aid station captain is carefully following the directions to mix up a cooler full of drink. By exposing your system to stronger solutions of drink during periodic training sessions, you'll be taking a step toward preventing the possibility of gastrointestinal distress on the day of the race.

9. **Load up on energy in the days before the race.** Studies show that consuming a high-carbohydrate diet (75 to 90 percent of calories from carbs) will fill up your liver and muscle glycogen stores for the race. Endurance sports scientist and author Dr. Timothy Noakes advises taking in approximately 500 grams of carbs each day during this period. Studies have also shown that following such a protocol can boost an athlete's exercise output—operating at 70 percent aerobic capacity (VO_2 max)—by 12 percent over athletes who eat a normal diet over these same three pre-effort days.

10. **Salt your food.** In conjunction with carbo-loading, make a point of including plenty of salt in your diet in the weeks leading up to your race, especially if you're preparing for

hot and muggy races like the Hawaii Ironman. This will help prepare your body for the hyponatremic effects that long races in strenuous conditions bring.

11. **Understand the correlation of race nutrition to race success.** Underestimating the value of this truth can be a catastrophe, while rigorously believing in it can be a competitive advantage. Training hard is important. Preparing your bike and equipment are both important activities. But in an Ironman competition you gain a solid advantage on your competition (be it the clock or your age-group peers) by treating nutrition as a sacred practice.

12. **Beware the side effects of caffeine.** Caffeine appears in a small percentage of gels and sports bars, and also in soda (for those athletes who gulp defizzed cola on race day). A moderate dose of the stimulant will give you a psychological charge and, according to certain studies, a physical boost as well. But don't let loopiness guide you into over-doing it.

13. **Don't allow yourself to neglect quality post-race nutrition.** Whether it's euphoria or despair, emotion often clouds your judgment of what you eat and drink or what you don't eat or drink after you cross the finish line. Remember that your body has just survived an exhaustive and brutal experience. Energy supplies are depleted and muscle structure has been damaged. Nutrients and minerals, especially salt, have been scraped out from every nook, and your body has been highway-robbed of it's most critical substance: water. Thus, the speed and proficiency of how your body repairs itself can be greatly aided by smart post-race nutrition.

14. **Don't skip breakfast.** The purpose of the pre-race breakfast, best consumed two to three hours before the race, is to top off glycogen stores, some of which have been depleted during the night's fast. Once again, simple, easy-to-digest carbs (white toast, sports bars, jam) are perfect choices for this meal.

15. **Beware the magic bullet.** When you see an advertising blurb that says "Increases endurance 300 percent!" or promises to peel off five pounds a week, you have every right to be skeptical. As a matter of fact, the FDA does not regulate the advertising of foods that fit under the banner of "food supplements" and makers of such supplements have more room to operate with their claims. Here's the real magic bullet: you need water, salt, and calories, and you need them in forms that climb right back up and out.

ENERGY FOOD REVIEW

Bars

Grabber Energy Bar

Flavors: Apple Strawberry, Apple Apricot, Apple Raspberry, Wild Mountain Berry
Review: Easy to eat all-carbs treat. A high-speed, lactose-free way to spike your blood with sugar with minimal digestion hassles.

Nu Bar

Flavors: Peanut Butter Cup and Lemon Crème

Review: More of a protein bar than a carbohydrate supplement, which makes it a good choice for post-race recovery.

Gatorade Energy Bar

Flavors: Chocolate, Peanut Butter, Mixed Berry

Review: Produced with a light, waffery Rice Krispies treat–like consistency, the Gatorade Bar offers a 47-gram wallop of carbs.

You Are What You Eat Energy Bar

Flavors: Peanut Butter, Blueberry Almond, Apple Cinnamon, Chocolate Fudgy

Review: Lactose-free and very easy to eat, with a homemade-cookie feel.

MET-Rx

Protein Plus Flavors: Chocolate Roasted Peanut, Peanut Butter

MET-Rx Bar Flavors: Chocolate Chip Cookie Dough, Java Chip, Chocolate Graham Cracker Chip

Review: Outstanding for recovery purposes during hard training phases and after races. The Protein Plus bars serve up a hefty 32 grams of protein, more than twice the amount of carbohydrates in the bar.

MET-Rx Total Nutrition Drink Mix Flavors: Chocolate Peanut Butter, White Chocolate Mousse

Review: Great for post-workout recovery and for triathletes that are either too busy to put together complete meals throughout the day or have trouble getting enough protein for whatever reason.

Clif Bar

Clif Bar Flavors: Chocolate Chip Peanut Butter, Crunchy Peanut Butter, Cookies 'n' Cream, Carrot Cake

Luna Bar Flavors: Chocolate Pecan Pie, Nuts Over Chocolate, Lemon Zest, Trail Mix

Review: Clif Bars are dairy-free and feature antioxidants.

Endurox

Flavors: Tangy Orange, Fruit Punch

Review: Endurox is *loaded* with carbs, so using it following intense exercise is a good way to rapidly begin the process of recovery and refueling depleted glycogen stores.

PR*Bar

Flavors: Peanut Butter Berry, Bavarian Mint, Chocolate Peanut

Review: Yummy Bavarian Mint and the others include a substantial amount of protein as well as carbohydrates, so they work well as supplements for recovery, training, and racing.

Omni Nutraceuticals 151 Bar

Flavors: Peanut Butter Chocolate, Power Fruit, Chocolate Cappucino, Fruit Burst, Fabulous Fruit, Chocolate Raspberry

Review: Heavy in vitamins, antioxidants, and minerals, this bar is a good choice if you're trying to not only take in carbs and protein, but also a wide-angled package of nutritional supplementation.

Promax Bar

Flavors: Black Forest Cake, Chocolate Chip Cookie Dough, Chocolate Mint, Chocolate Peanut Crunch, Cookies 'n Cream, Double Fudge Brownie, Lemon, Nutty Butter Crisp, Honey Peanut

Review: SportsPharma, a cult favorite among triathletes, is a great post-exercise snack because it's loaded with protein.

Cheetah Bar

Flavors: Strawberry, Lemon, Peach Apricot

Review: Chewy, moist, and made with all-natural organic ingredients, this is one of the most easy-to-eat bars.

Balance Bar

Balance Outdoor: Honey Almond, Chocolate Crisp, Nut Berry, Crunchy Peanut

Balance Bar: Honey Peanut, Yogurt Honey Peanut, Chocolate

Balance+: Chocolate Banana Plus Antioxidants, Yogurt Berry Plus Ginkgo Biloba, Honey Peanut Plus Ginseng

Review: Balance Bars have developed a cult following both inside and outside the athletic community because they don't forget to make taste a priority. Lots of good flavors to choose from, but Honey Peanut won *Triathlete Magazine*'s taste test hands down.

PowerBar

Flavors: Apple, Original, Chocolate, Mocha, Banana, Malt Nut, Apple Cinnamon, Wild Berry, Peanut Butter, Oatmeal Raisin, Vanilla Crisp, Chocolate Peanut Butter

PowerBar Harvest Flavors: Blueberry, Peanut Butter Chocolate Chip, Cherry Crunch, Apple Crisp, Chocolate, Strawberry

PowerBar Essentials Flavors: Chocolate, Peanut Butter Chocolate, Berries & Yogurt, Chocolate Raspberry Truffle

Review: Back in the old days, the only problem with PowerBars was that if you chowed down on them on a consistent basis, you eventually became exhausted by the three flavors that were available. Obviously, that problem has been stamped out. In the "original" category of flavors alone, PowerBar has added seven distinct flavors to the chocolate, malt nut, and wild berry that we used to endlessly rotate.

Energy Drinks

Champion Nutrition Revenge Sport

Review: Good in the sodium department and plenty of carbohydrates.

Gatorade

Traditional Gatorade Flavors: Lemon-Lime, Orange, Fruit Punch, Lemon Ice, Citrus Cooler, Grape Watermelon, Tropical Burst, Mandarina, Cherry Rush, Strawberry Kiwi, Cool Blue Raspberry, Midnight Thunder

Gatorade Frost Flavors: Alpine Snow, Glacier Freeze, Whitewater Splash, Riptide Rush

Gatorade Fierce Flavors: Fierce Melon, Fierce Lime

Review: Gatorade continues to adhere to their no-bull program, producing a drink that supplies energy in a liquid solution in scientifically well-supported proportions of carbohydrates, water, and sodium. No "secret" ingredients necessary. The cool thing is that they make a rainbow of flavors, all of which taste good.

SoBe

SoBe Powerline: Drive, Edge, Energy, Power, Wisdom

Lizard Fuel (before exercise): Cherry-Citrus, Fruit Punch, Blackberry, Strawberry Banana

Lizard Blizzard (before exercise): Dairy-based, with a tropical fruit flavor.

Review: New on the sports drink market is SoBe, and the spectrum of flavors and ingredients is as out of the ordinary as the names. Fun stuff and very tasty.

ProLyte Sports Drink

Flavors: Electric Lemon Lime, Citrus Buzz, Tropical Rocket, Racin' Raspberry

Review: Good formula and good selection of flavors.

Omni Nutraceuticals

Beyond Endurance Stamina & Energy Shake: Rich Chocolate

Smart Fuel

BUZ RN (before exercise): Chocolate

WarpAIDE (during exercise): Wild Wildberry, Tangy Lemon, Mellow Mandarin

Bio FIX (after exercise): Peach Mango, Orange-Pineapple, Raspberry Lemon

Review: Smart Fuel offers a complete sports drink program with a nice array of flavors to choose from.

Gels

Why chew? Energy gels give you some of the nutrients of food with the convenience of a slurp. Most provides simple sugar for quick bursts of enegy. Others have extra protein for recovery.

Clif Shot

Flavors: Cocoa Peanut, Mocha Mocha, Razz Sorbet, Peanut Buzz, Viva Vanilla
Review: Very zesty mix of flavors. Vanilla is our favorite.

GU

Flavors: Chocolate Outrage, Vanilla Bean, Orange Blast, Banana Blitz, Tri Berry
Review: We figure that Chocolate Outrage is the most widely preferred gel on the market. "Tastes like chocolate frosting!" said one tester.

Jog Mate

Flavors: Chocolate, Vanilla
Review: The gel that is designed for after you've crossed the finish line. Laden with protein. The chocolate reminds us of pudding.

Squeezy

Flavors: Pineapple, Grape, Vanilla.
Review: Offered in large bottles as well as packet form, so you can use it with flasks.

14 WAYS TO FUEL ON THE BIKE

Fueling on the bike is a key factor in strong training and racing, especially during events or training sessions over 90 minutes, and I've seen no one explain it as well as Rebecca Marks Rudy, MS. She says the bike leg is a golden opportunity to refuel from the swim and prepare for the run, and it's easy to see why. Since your stomach isn't jostling around and you can actually carry a fair amount of food along, the bike is really the only chance all race that you'll have to eat solid nutrition and lots of it. And the bike leg, according to a study by Jeukendrup et al. in 2005, may be the best opportunity to ingest fluids.

Of course, says Rudy, preparation helps. Training rides and early season races are occasions to master the mechanics of fueling on the bike, such as reaching into a cycling jersey to grab a snack and eating with one hand while controlling your bike with the other. Here's some ways to facilitate the process:

1. Keep the snack in the pocket nearest to your retrieving hand; avoid burying the fuel under spare tubes and tools.

2. Open wrappers before your ride. Or place a bagel, crackers, fig cookies, or pretzels into sandwich baggies; if using Ziplocs, keep the bags unlocked for easy access.

3. Carry bars and gels in a top tube Bento Box or Aero Pocket that sits between your aerobars, especially for longer events, including a half or full Ironman.

4. For shorter distances, it is possible to haul all you need directly on your bike. Use electrical tape to attach pieces of snacks (like Clif Bar bites) to your top tube.

5. Stick PowerBars length wise around the tube.

6. Tape a gel pack to your top tube or aerobars by the tab, which you will want to tear just slightly; the gel pack, when released from the tape, is already conveniently opened. (Bring one extra in case the pack does land on the road; during a race you won't want to take the time to retrieve the hapless gel.)

7. Attach a gel flask holder to your bike; the flask is refillable with your gel of choice (for example, Hammer Gel from Hammer Nutrition is available in multiple-serving jugs).

8. Beware chocolate and yogurt coatings; they tend to create an undesirable mess if exposed to sweat, rain, or intense heat. If the snack falls apart or becomes too unappealing to eat you could miss out on the energy necessary for optimal performance.

9. Get easy-to-chew foods, since your increased rate of breathing might hinder your ability to chew. Some foods melt in your mouth more easily than others. A Nutri-Grain cereal bar may work well for one person while a Quaker Chewy Granola Bar might be better for another. Establish what works for you, preferably during training sessions, not the race.

10. Rely on liquid fuel for sprint or Olympic distance races, using a couple of bottles mounted to your frame, saddle, seat post, or between your aerobars. In the latter, fluid is consumed through a straw, allowing you to maintain your "aero" position while drinking.

11. Practice refilling your aerobar-mounted bottle with solution from a bottle stored elsewhere or from one acquired in an exchange. Avoid doing so while descending at high speeds.

12. Select a drink that has 5 to 8 percent carbohydrate solution, such as a Gatorade. 10 percent or higher concentration (straight orange juice, for instance) may cause gastrointestinal discomfort. The high sugar content can cause a slower release of fluid into your intestines and delay absorption.

13. Carbohydrate remains your best source of energy for training and racing. The American College of Sports Medicine recommends ingesting 60 to 70 grams of carbohydrate per hour, or up to one gram of carbohydrate per minute of exercise. Certainly, energy bars and sports drinks, as well as hybrid gel packs, are marketed to enhance performance. In addition to providing easily digested carbohydrates (with various combinations of glucose, glucose polymers, sucrose, and fructose), they often have additional nutrients that are beneficial to athletes, such as sodium

and potassium. These electrolytes are minerals that, among other functions, help regulate normal body fluid levels, acid-base balance, maintain blood pressure, and assist muscle contraction. Consuming fuel—whether as sports drinks, energy bars or gel packs—with sodium and potassium during endurance events is beneficial because electrolyte balance can be disrupted through sweat loss.

14. Eat some real foods, which often naturally provide performance-enhancing nutrients. After all, athletes lived, competed, and excelled long before the arrival of energy bars! The tables below compare select nutrient values of different fuel sources, with examples of foods, fluids, and gels.

Whichever combination of fuel you decide is right for you is a product of trial and, most likely, some error. So, just as you are diligent to log endurance miles, master dismounts, and rehearse transitions, continue to practice your nutrition. Remember that you are not only eating to train, you are also training to eat.

Sample Food Sources

Source	Calories	Carbohydrate (g)	Sodium (mg)	Potassium (mg)
Banana (7 in)	105	27	—	422
Clif Bar	240	40	150	256
Fig Newtons (4)	240	40	240	160
Peanut Butter Sandwich*	340	51	400	112
Pretzels (2 oz)	215	44	972	83

* Made with 2 slices of whole wheat bread, 1 tbsp peanut butter, and 1 tbsp honey.

Sample Fluid Sources

Source	Calories	Carbohydrate (g)	Sodium (mg)	Potassium (mg)
Cytomax powder (1 scoop)	95	20	100	110
Gatorade (16 oz)	120	30	192	53
Orange Juice (8 oz)	110	26	3	496
Powerade (16 oz)	144	38	56	64
Hammer HEED (1 scoop)	100	25	62	16
Accelerade (1 scoop)	120	21	190	65

Sample Gel Sources

Source	Calories	Carbohydrate (g)	Sodium (mg)	Potassium (mg)
Clif Shot	100	25	40	30
GU	100	20	55	40
Hammer Gel	90	22	45	not available
PowerBar Gel	120	28	200	20
Accel Gel	90	20	95	40

THE ESSENTIAL PRE-SWIM WARM-UP

Most triathletes at some point have had the experience of good intentions standing on the beach, but as soon as the horn sounds and you're swallowed by the pack, getting kicked or hit in your face, head, arms, and every part of your body, you get thrown completely off course, mentally and physically, and shrink back to avoid the chaos. Though your progress in the pool is encouraging, swimming with the pack is so stressful that you can't employ the skills you've been building.

The key to the entire swim can be the *tone* you set in the initial 100 to 200 meters by remaining contained in the midst of what can feel like aquatic anarchy. Even after 32 years of open water racing experience and dozens of age group wins, swimming guru Terry Laughlin says he still finds it nerve-wracking. "It's easy to be shaken from the physical and mental state in which I know I swim my best," he says. "With the advantage of extensive seasoning and deep neuromuscular imprinting I've learned how to regain that groove, but it can take a hundred or more strokes to find it. A less comfortable or experienced athlete could easily find himself floundering helplessly for most of the swim leg without a plan for gaining and maintaining control." The tips below are what Laughlin has found has worked for him. More information on his swim methods can be found at www.TotalImmersion.net or by calling 1-800-609-7946.

Warm-up

I find the warm-up swim essential for several reasons:

1. **Course reconnaissance:** I always swim to at least the first turn buoy, and often some distance along where the course goes after that, checking for sight lines and how the course and buoys will appear while I'm swimming. Are there landmarks I can use if the buoy is hard to see because of glare, waves, or swell? Is there a sweep moving parallel to shore? If there's a westward sweep, for instance, I know I need to position myself to the east at the start.

2. **Bottom configuration:** How far will I have to run and porpoise before swimming? Are there pebbles or shells? Where are the waves breaking? All this info goes into my mental rehearsal.

3. **Planning my exit:** Swimming from the final buoy back toward shore, I familiarize myself with how the finish line/chute appears when I make the final turn, so I can line up accurately. I also learn where I might be able to catch a wave and/or at what point my hands will scrape the bottom so I can get to my feet and start high-stepping through the shallows. I also check to see if there are visual cues such as how the bottom appears through my goggles, which will alert me that I'm approaching the finish.

4. **Tune-ups:** Everything I've mentioned thus far is strategic preparation. The physical preparation is equally important. If the first buoy is 50 to 100 meters from shore, I'll likely swim back and forth between it and the shallows three or more times. The first 200 meters or so, I'm just loosening. After that, it's specific rehearsal. This means swimming short bursts of about ten strokes with exactly the power and tempo I plan to use in the first 100 to 200 meters of the race. The effect of this is both to prime my muscles and nervous system for the task they'll be executing in a few minutes and to imprint my brain with the same information. That really helps me find the feel I'm seeking to remain effective in the middle of what likely feels like turmoil to others. Having no natural speed, I have to find every edge I can.

5. **Staying ready:** I stay in the water, swimming easily back and forth near the start line until called out to line up. Again, I find it much easier to maintain a sense of calm and control by swimming easily, and continuing to *groove* the smooth feeling I want by doing that than when I'm milling about on the beach with everyone else. Sprinters like their muscles really rested for a burst of power. Distance swimmers do better when they stay loose and warm.

The Start

"In past years I avoided the crowd when I lined up for the start," says Laughlin. "Now, I'm swimming stronger and faster and feel more ready to mix it up and race for a better position in the first 100 meters. But I wouldn't expect most triathletes would be comfortable or able to establish good control in that environment." So now he counsels most to start at the edge of the pack to give yourself space in the first 100 meters to find your most comfortable and effective stroking pattern.

Unless the swim is less than 400 meters, the race won't be decided in those first 100 meters. If it's at least one kilometer, take your time at the start and focus on establishing control. Blend into or follow the pack at a slow speed. Stroke with unhurried overlapping strokes with one hand always extended in front to ward off thrashing legs. Swim with a compact, high-elbow recovery to protect your space from the side. The more chaotic it gets around you, the more you should focus on control and a smooth, firm grip. If your goggles get knocked askew, roll onto your back and kick easily while adjusting them.

You can also save time and energy by not repeatedly looking for the first buoy. The whole pack is heading in that direction and virtually everyone else *will* be looking. Just keep your head down, follow the energy and bubbles, and get your bearings as you breathe to both sides. If there are swimmers for some distance on either side, you're going the right way. It's a given that you're going to look at some point, but try to control the instinct to look frequently. Take another 6 to 10 strokes after the instinct hits, to develop a bit more trust in your ability to stay on course without looking frequently. Every avoided peek is a bit more energy and control moving you toward your goal.

As you approach the first buoy, there will be a piranha pack fighting for the closest position. Swim 5 to 10 yards outside to avoid them, take a good look at where everyone is heading, and then fall in with them at a comfortable pace.

Find Your Place... and Pace

After you pass that first buoy, you'll see quite a few caps ahead of you—that's good as it gives you a better target to follow. Aim for the middle of the cluster and then put your head down for 20 strokes before sighting again. If you're behind other swimmers and feel as if your pace is comfortable, stay there, saving energy by following their draft and letting them sight for you. If you lose focus, begin counting strokes, in sets of 20, to occupy your mind. Swim more quietly and with slower strokes than anyone in your vicinity. This will quiet your mind and save energy.

Finish

Unlike in a pool where your lap count tells you how far you've gone, in open water you lose your sense of time and distance, so continue to swim conservatively. If you do whatever it takes to stay calm and to swim economically, you'll pass many swimmers almost without effort because in open water, as in road races, most people start too fast. Once you jog out of the water, the real race starts. Enjoy it; you should have plenty of energy to ride and run your best.

15 HAWAII IRONMAN DOS AND DON'TS

The Hawaii Ironman race week can wear you out with pressure, tension, anxiety, nerves, stress, jitters, jumps, sleeplessness, and more. I know; I did the race once. But you don't have to let all of the stress get to you. The following dos and don'ts will help you arrive at the starting line less than completely frazzled.

1. **Do have a carefully written nutrition plan.** Veterans of Hawaii know well that a single nutrition error will derail your race like Godzilla toying with a cable car. Dr. Jeff Zachwieja, PhD, is a senior scientist at the Gatorade Sports Science Institute who has

made frequent visits to the Hawaii Ironman and has sound advice for the newcomer. "Triathletes spend such amazing amounts of time training," he says. "If they only spent a fraction of the time they spend on training to plan their nutrition for an Ironman, they'd avoid so much trouble." Just ask any of the successful elites what the "secret" is to Hawaii, and in most cases they'll tell you it's about getting and keeping down food, water, sports drinks, and salt before and during the race.

2. **Do rent *The Blues Brothers*.** There's nothing like watching Jake and Elwood drive the Bluesmobile through the Nazis to release the bite that pre-race nerves like to sink into you. Other comedies might also work, but surely not as well.

3. **Do put on flip-flops immediately after you finish your morning swim.** It's easy to get lulled into pre-race bull sessions with your buddies after you've finished your swim in the bay. But get some flip-flops on, or take a chance burning the bottoms of your feet while idly standing around on the pavement; unless you like having the worst case of hot foot imaginable during the hardest bike leg of your life. I know this because this is exactly what happened to me in 2000.

4. **Do go on the Body Glove Snorkel and Dolphin Cruise.** It's great. The Body Glove boat takes off from the Kailua Pier both in the morning and again in the afternoon for a short cruise up along the coast of the island. First you'll spot a pod of dolphins, and then you set anchor in a delightful snorkeling spot in Pawai Bay. They have all the equipment, and lounging is the theme of the day. You'll feel like you're a million miles away from Kona (www.BodyGloveHawaii.com).

5. **Don't freak out and join a cult.** Not too long ago an Oakland Raider, in the preceding days before the Super Bowl, decided it was a good idea to go into Tijuana and see how much tequila he could drink. This is an extreme case, but the point is keep an eye on yourself. The pressure, the atmosphere, and the adrenaline that encapsulate you in Kona can subconsciously spur you to do something stupid to sabotage your race. You see, *you* want to do the Hawaii Ironman. However, deep inside your brain is a more sensible mechanism that prefers survival. Beware.

6. **Do visit the Hilton Waikoloa Village.** A dreamy place to visit out on the Queen K to get away from the noise of Kona. The Hilton has it all. If you have kids, they'll love the dolphin show and you'll join them playing in the coolest swimming pool on earth. They have restaurants that serve extraordinarily healthy food, and the Hilton is into the race: in years past they've held Q&A seminars with athletes like Luc Van Lierde and Lisa Bentley (www.HiltonWaikoloaVillage.com).

7. **Don't use your special needs bag for bananas.** There will be about one million bananas to choose from at aid stations. Use your special needs bag for a gel that won't be offered or your favorite candy bar or your pet rock.

8. **Don't avoid salt in your diet.** You are not the person and this is not the time to eliminate salt from you diet. Salt, now more than ever, is your best friend. Liberally salt your food in the days leading up to the race so that you'll be better armed for the insane amount of sweating that lies ahead.

9. **Do get a couples massage at the Fairmont Orchid.** Another lovely getaway not far from Kona, the Fairmont Orchid may be one of the most romantic spots in the world to take your loyal, loving, and ever-patient spouse, that life partner of yours who has been putting up with dozens of weekend mega-brick training sessions. Treat yourselves to the couples massage in their waterfall-laden "Spa Without Walls" (www.Fairmont.com).

10. **Don't arrive at check-ins late.** There will be a long line, and you'll be late for dinner, going nuts that you're standing on feet that you're trying to save up for the big day. Plus you'll be more apt to suffer a brain freeze and put the running shoes in the cycling bag. Don't torture yourself. Get to these things as early as you can.

11. **Don't drag race down Alii Drive on the Thursday before the race.** It happens every year. Pumped up athletes throw their best race away because they can't help from showing off their fitness on the runway that is Alii Drive. Our advice? Wear a heart rate monitor and blinders and make sure your taper jogs and bike sessions are short and easy.

12. **Do eat a pre-race breakfast.** The best way to trigger your body's fat-burning powers is to eat a low-glycemic, high-carb breakfast—about two hours before the race—that is easily digestible. Not an easy find, but one thing to check out is the new Elite Performance Pancake & Waffle Mix (www.ElitePerformance1.com). Formulated by a triathlete working with dieticians, the pancakes are tasty, digest quickly, and will work for you the whole day. You need to use sugar-free syrup to keep it a low-glycemic meal, but when you keep it low-glycemic, the insulin response is tamed and your body engages fat-burning earlier in the race (rather than tearing through glycogen stores).

13. **Do wear a hat during the race.** The Kona sun is a killer, and you can fill your hat with ice at an aid station and turn it into a remote refrigerator. Pick a light color, like white, that will reflect the sun. For that matter, pick a race outfit that isn't black (black sponges up the heat from the sun—just what you need). Paula Newby-Fraser might be able to race well in black, but if you want to get away with it too, become Paula Newby-Fraser.

14. **Don't rush the transitions.** Saving a few seconds by rushing through a transition area is as wise as grocery shopping at a vending machine. By being attentive to your body's needs with Vaseline, equipment, food, and sunblock, you ultimately shave away at least a few of the minutes of time that would have been spent hobbling along and swearing at yourself.

15. **Don't get bummed out if it doesn't go perfectly.** Why? Because it never goes perfectly in Hawaii. Ask six-time Hawaii Ironman champion Mark Allen. He'll tell you no matter how completely he prepared, the day always threw him a knuckleball. Even on the luckiest of days at least one thing goes wrong. The key is to keep your cool, get through it the best you can, and recall what a weird, wonderful thing it is to be racing in the Hawaii Ironman.

13

OLD DOGS, NEW TRICKS

EIGHT TIPS TO HELP OLDER TRIATHLETES FIGHT OFF THE RAVAGING FORCES OF AGE

The performance most savored by the great Dave Scott was not one of his six Hawaii Ironman titles. Scott says he most relishes his fifth place finish, at the sober age of 42, in 1996. An empty-legged 4:49:55 bike ride had left him struggling well behind 20th place, but a 2:45:20 marathon catapulted the legend past an army of younger and arguably more talented athletes. Out-splitting the likes of Greg Welch, Thomas Hellriegel, and up-and-coming Peter Reid (winner Luc Van Lierde was the only top-10 finisher who ran faster), Scott fired up the hearts and hopes of older triathletes around the world.

A look at the World Championship record books show how triathletes are drilling holes in the walls of age-related decline. In her late 50s, Cherie Gruenfeld cracked 12 hours at the 1999 Hawaii Ironman. That same year, Duncan Thomas set the 50 to 54 record with a 9:44:13.

Possibly the most remarkable age-group performance ever was Bob Scott, 71, who raced an astonishing 12:59:02 in 2001. While all senior triathletes have the salty Walt Stack to thank for his pioneering efforts in the early days of the Hawaii Ironman, Walt's 26:20:00 (at the age of 73) wasn't even half as fast.

If you're beginning to segue from your 30s to your 40s—or beyond—the first thing to learn from the elders is mindset. Dismiss notions that all will soon be lost. Know that ultradistance events favor the temperament and accumulated strength of a veteran athlete. By studying the effects of aging and working aggressively to diminish them with training and dietary solutions, you can stake your claim in triathlon's attack on the aging barrier. Following are some suggestions to get you started.

1. **It's not enough to obey your thirst.** As we get older, our sense of thirst diminishes. Because of the sweaty nature of the sport, triathletes must especially address this need. Our blood, for example, is more than 80 percent water. We need about two gallons a day when we're training hard. Even a modest level of dehydration is severely detrimental to performance. Now more than ever, don't let thirst be your guide.

2. **Hydrate with fresh fruit.** Hydrating doesn't just mean guzzling Aquafina. Two or more pieces of fruit at each meal packs a hydrating punch as well as drenching your systems in anti-aging vitamins, antioxidants, and phytonutrients. Add berries and

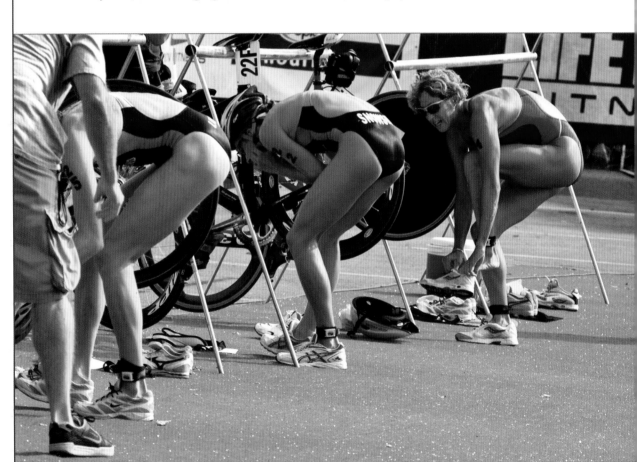

melons to the standard ration of apples, oranges, and bananas. You'll back up your hydration efforts and aid your recovery to workouts.

3. **Stretch your calves.** The normal human being has to fend off the hardening effects of aging on tendons and ligaments. The serious triathlete also needs to spend time worrying about retaining a degree of suppleness in the muscles. Dave Scott, who performs stretches throughout the day, begs the athletes he coaches to stretch. If you've never made stretching and flexibility a staple of your training, now's the time to wedge it in. Triathlon legend and New Zealand–based coach Scott Molina says that in addition to focusing on the hamstrings, glutes, quadriceps, lower back, and shoulder muscles, pay special attention to the calf muscles. Increased range of motion in the calves prevents injury and enhances your speed and power.

4. **Don't back off from intensity.** Aerobic capacity backslides about 9 percent per decade after the age of 25. Part of this is aging that we can't do anything about, another part isn't. Exercise makes a huge difference. Additionally, author and coach Joe Friel has noted that older athletes aren't as enthusiastic about speed workouts as the young ones. "They tend to shy away from high intensity, and opt for the longer races," Friel says. Consider this observation a weakness in your age group competitors that you

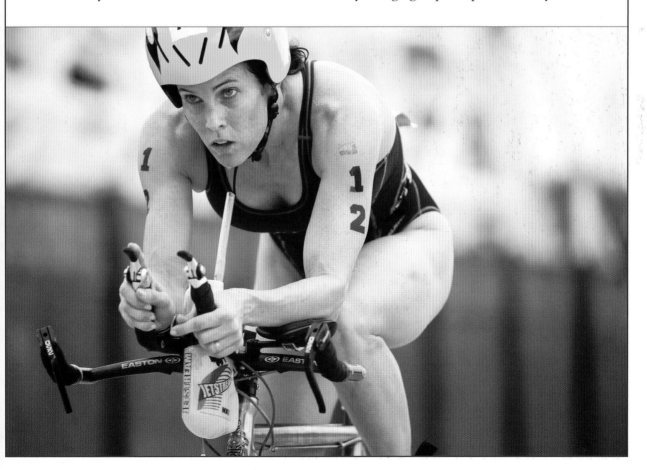

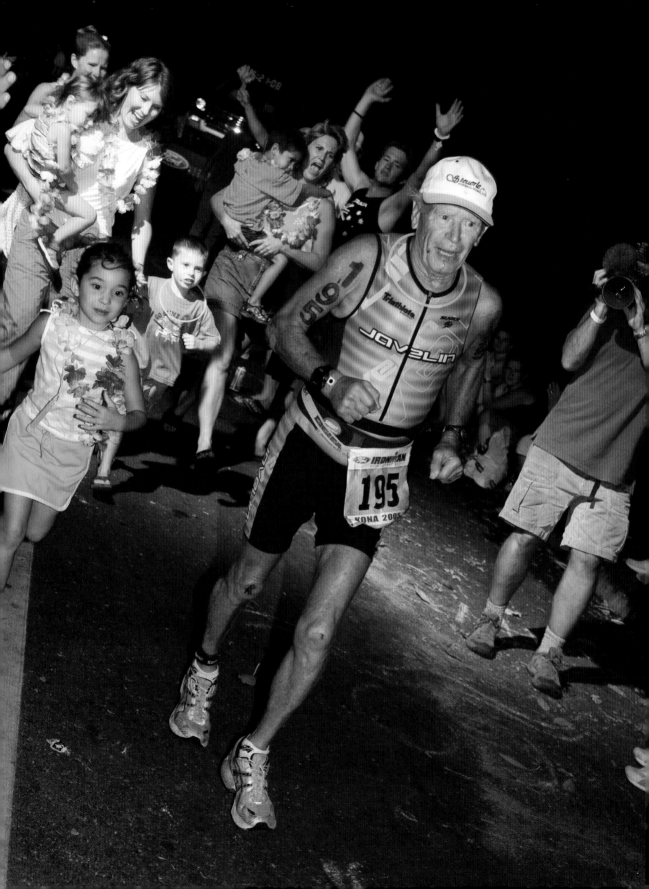

can prey upon. By mixing in tempo, hill, and interval workouts, you'll maximize your aerobic and anaerobic systems, despite the natural decline.

5. **Strength train twice a week.** Those who don't get to the weight room can suffer a 30 percent loss of strength and 40 percent loss of muscle mass between the ages of 20 and 70. Not only do you lose power, but basal metabolism slows, making it easier to replace rock hard abs with a beer gut. Weight training is the remedy, and no one has exploited this antidote to power loss better than Dave Scott. In addition to helping him achieve high levels of performance in his 40s, Scott has long maintained that weight training heartily improves a marathon run after a 112-mile bike ride.

6. **Break out of ruts.** One of the fundamental principles of training—stressing our systems with a workout will be rewarded with positive adaptations—has a clause that can work against us as the years go by. If we do the same workouts and training routines season after season, our bodies will get amazingly good at the workouts and routines, but overall performance will slump. Do 4 × 800 meters as your key track workout every week for a long time, and you get so efficient at the specific intervals and rest periods that you lose the cream of the training effect. What do you do? Figure this loophole into your training. Switch things up with a variety of workouts and schedules. Try new types of workouts and new types of programs. Our bodies respond powerfully to being shocked. Go to a new triathlon camp, try out an off-road triathlon, mix in some new distances. You'll have fun and spark fresh progress.

7. **Lean on your technique.** The negative adaptations will, in the long run, snatch away a measure of your power and speed. However, some of this loss can be counterbalanced with gains in technique and efficiency. Hire a running coach to study your mechanics and prescribe drills. Adding numbers to your stride count and inches to your stride length will see your marathon times plummet. Renew your commitment to technique in the pool—it's everything in the swim. Better technique means you get out of the drink having used less energy, which means more for later. Go to a triathlon or bike camp and get your bike position tweaked toward perfection. Be like Lance Armstrong, and master your pedaling technique with drills and analysis (bike camps and CompuTrainer SpinScans will help you accomplish this). Armstrong "mashed" the pedals in his youth, channeling his raw force almost solely into the downward stroke. You don't win Tour de France titles this way, it's too wasteful. Now his stroke is as smooth as checkered silk.

8. **Send the kids off to college.** It's not much of a joke. One reason we're seeing more triathletes in their 50s prancing through Ironmans like they are 22 is because they have more time to train. If you can't afford to retire early, or the kids are a little young to march off to Yale, see if you can't at least treat yourself to one season free of too much external responsibility. Take the time and train like you're Heather Fuhr or Luc Van Lierde. You may truly surprise yourself.

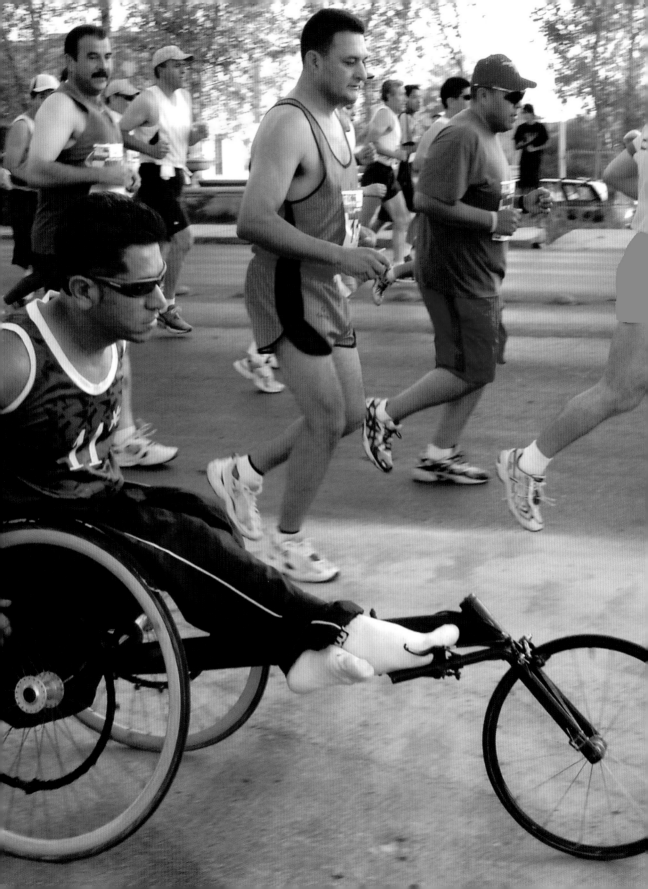

14
GET
INSPIRED

NEED INSPIRATION? SEE WHY WHEELCHAIR-BOUND CARLOS MOLEDA AND DAVID BAILEY MADE FOR THE GREATEST RIVALRY IN TRIATHLON HISTORY

Spinal cord injuries usually occur from a traumatic impact that breaks a vertebra. When discs or bone fragments rupture spinal cord tissue, the initial wave of damage can shred neural cells and crush axons. Heavy bleeding can swell the tissues within the spinal canal, cutting off blood and oxygen flow to other regions of the cord. The drop in blood pressure can impede self-regulation systems and lead to spinal shock. Neurologists believe this happens in half of all spinal cord injuries. Spinal shock disrupts communication between the brain and the body. Essentially, the first blow of the accident is the start, and in the hours, days, and weeks that follow, the damage grows. Problems throughout the body can include paralysis.

Collision causes most spinal cord injuries, although certain diseases, like cancer, can also be the source. Approximately 50 percent of spinal cord injuries in the United States occur in auto

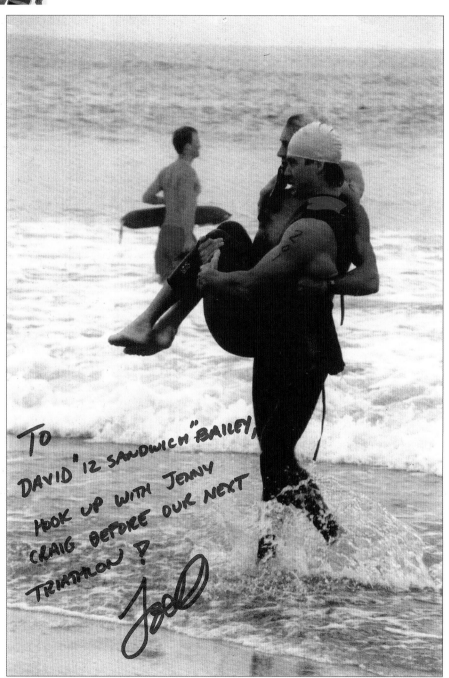

To
DAVID "12 SANDWICH" BAILEY,
HOOK UP WITH JENNY
CRAIG BEFORE OUR NEXT
TRIATHLON?
Joel

and motorcycle accidents, about 22 percent result from falls, 15 percent from violent acts like knife wounds or gunshots, and 8 percent from sports accidents.

Despite how tough it is to rebound from spinal cord injuries—in addition to enormous physical adaptation, doctors list denial, grief, and depression as common obstacles in recovery—wheelchair athletes have thrived in sports since shortly after World War II, when the Stoke Mandeville Games were held on the opening day of the 1948 London Olympics. The brainchild of Dr. Ludwig Guttman, the first director of the National Spinal Injuries Centre in Britain, Guttman used athletics because traditional methods of rehabilitation were falling short. The Stoke Mandeville Games evolved into the Paralympic Games that exist today.

After being paralyzed, the journey to the starting line of an endurance event is long, painful, and complicated. It can take months of healing and rehabilitation time to simply develop the strength to live through a basic life routine. Remarkably, in the early to mid-1990s, the question of whether a wheelchair triathlete could finish the Hawaii Ironman was tested and resolved. In 1996, John Maclean was the first wheelchair triathlete to complete the Ironman in regulation time.

David Bailey was paralyzed in a motorcycle accident in 1987. Carlos Moleda was shot in 1989. They would meet for the first time in a half Ironman in 1997, a precursor to their three-year rivalry at the Hawaii Ironman, a rivalry that transcended the disabilities that might have defined them. From the first cannon blast, any question of whether they could finish the race was dismissed. It was competition to win, a boxing match fueled by hatred of losing. The sport has seen legendary rivalries before: Dave Scott and Mark Allen, Paula Newby-Fraser and Erin Baker. But a strong case can be made that Bailey versus Moleda was the greatest one of all.

Having started out at the age of 10 on a 60cc Yamaha, David Bailey's motocross potential revealed itself when he won the 1978 250cc Amateur National Championship at 17. As he tells the story, a crucial moment in his first years of struggle to break in as a pro occurred in 1981. He had borrowed his mom's Toyota Celica and, lacking a trailer, took the front wheel off of his motorbike so he could bolt the forks to the car's hitch. In the Celica, wedged full of gear and a gas can, with a brake light dangling from the back of his Kawasaki, Bailey proceeded to drive from his home in Virginia to a race in Denver where he hoped to qualify for pro nationals.

In the race, Bailey was leading when a competitor's crash on another stretch of the track plowed through hay bales and "center-punched" him, breaking a rib and ending his race. "I drove all that way to race three laps," he says. Despite the pain of the rib, he piled everything back in the car, hitched up his bike into the endless wheelie, and began driving back to the East Coast that night, leaving the Rocky Mountains behind him.

While driving, something in the night caught Bailey's eye. "It looked like a cloud," he recalled in an interview with Competitor.com. "I pulled over and just stared at it. It was the Milky Way." Under the starry sweep of sky, Bailey examined his motocross dream. "I made up my mind. This is what I want to do. This is what I'm willing to do. *I'm going to do whatever it takes.*" In less than two years, he would sign a coveted deal with Honda to be on their factory team. Not only had he made it, his career soared. In his eight-year career, Bailey collected 30 AMA victories and was eventually inducted into the Motorcycle Hall of Fame in 1999.

Held on dirt courses erected within major sports arenas, supercross races are known for their steep jumps and demanding obstacles. In a 1986 supercross event held in Anaheim, California, Bailey got into a dogfight with Ricky Johnson, a Honda teammate, in a race that is considered one of the greatest in motocross history. Bailey and Johnson exploited slim tangents and openings as they lapped other riders, repeatedly stealing the lead from each other. The tension of the duel lit up the fans, and Bailey says he gauged Johnson's moves by crowd reaction. Endurance became a factor after 10 laps of the 19-lap race. Johnson later said he went anaerobic at about lap 12 and hung on for five more laps before giving in to Bailey's pressure. "My lungs were bleeding," Johnson recalled in an interview with RacerXill.com on the 20th anniversary of the race. "I was seeing dots at the end. I gave it everything I had. And I knew I was going to have to do that every single weekend for the whole series. I was just thinking about what it was going to take to beat him."

The race displayed the essence of Bailey's talent. A good dirt-bike racer knows the intricacies of a course and breaks each lap into concise segments, mustering complete concentration on mastering each increment, one at a time, before moving on to the next. According to his longtime trainer and best friend, former professional triathlete Todd Jacobs, Bailey brought to motocross an exceptional intelligence in seeing and handling a course. "David used a natural genius he possessed for finding the cleanest, most efficient lines," Jacobs says. For instance, Bailey pioneered a technique using the brake while airborne during a jump to tip the front wheel and sweeten the landing, reducing impact and retaining speed. Jacobs, now a trainer for

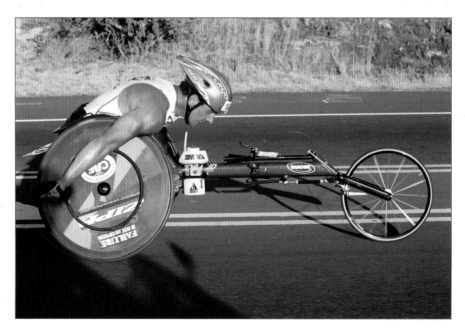

Bakke-Svensson/Ironman

motocross riders, says Bailey could plumb a course during the few minutes allowed for warm-up at a level well beyond his competition. In the duel between Bailey and Johnson, Bailey showed an uncanny ability to guide a motorcycle on the finest of angles and lines, before, during, and after jumps. When Johnson's final two stabs at the lead were instantly reversed, the viewer got a sense not only of Bailey's skill but his raw desire to win—to do, as he declared earlier in his life, "whatever it takes."

"It wasn't Ricky Johnson" motivating him that day, Bailey says. "It was the idea of someone being able to dominate me. I hated it."

In 1987 at a preseason event in Lake Huron, California, at a time when Bailey was riding at speeds experts in the sport believed were unprecedented, Bailey's life took the severe turn that would ultimately guide him into triathlon. The weather was overcast and Bailey, as he tells it, didn't want to race. "It was a lousy day," he says. In part of a bid to try and get it over with, Bailey decided to try and get two jumps over with at the same time. It didn't work and he went over the handlebars, and the bike followed him to the ground. The crash would leave Bailey paraplegic.

Well before the accident, Bailey had become a rabid fan of triathlon. On his honeymoon in Hawaii with his wife, Gina, in 1986, he was in Kona to watch the race in person. In addition to pioneering technique in motocross, he was also one of the first to use triathlon as an ancillary

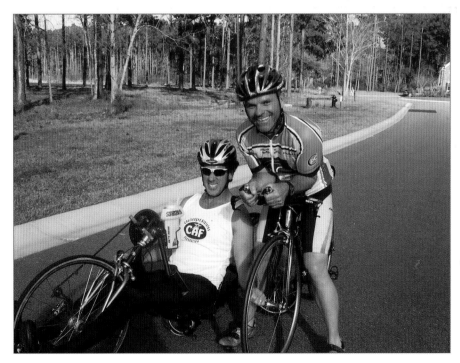

Courtesy of Andrew Chafer

form of training to improve performance. Outlasting Ricky Johnson was one example of how this paid off.

In the two years following the injury, Bailey obsessed on finding a way to walk again. Whether it was word of experimental surgery, mental imagery, or medicinal herbs, he pursued it. While he received warm encouragement and support from friends and loved ones, Bailey says it was straight talk from Jeff Spencer, a former Olympic cyclist who was working as a fitness consultant for the Honda racing team, that helped him. As Bailey ticked off the various methods he was chasing to regain use of his legs, Spencer repeated the question, "What if it doesn't work?" Bailey says this woke him up. "I realized I was going to have to deal with it, now, head on. I had never asked myself, 'What can I learn from this?' I had been so busy trying to get back on my feet. In life, we all have our time when we have to deal with problems. They can shape us, teach us patience, resolve, purpose, and faith."

Bailey's journey back into athletic competition began in his wheelchair, going up and down his driveway. In the early 1990s, he would meet another straight talker, Jacobs, and the two would develop a lifelong friendship through which they shared knowledge. From Bailey, Jacobs received an education in the art of motocross and the art of patience; from Jacobs, Bailey was able to learn from the depths and experiences of a former professional triathlete who had trained with and competed against the best—the likes of Mark Allen, Dave Scott, Scott Tinley, and Scott Molina.

"He kept pestering me about triathlons," Jacobs says. "He wanted to know all about the Ironman. He'd followed it for a long time, and could recite the ABC telecasts. One day I said, 'Let's just do one.'"

They picked a relatively low-key event, the Carlsbad Triathlon. "It grew to be an obsession," Jacobs says. "I realized the process was helping him save his life. It was his reentry into being a man."

Whatever challenge triathlon poses to an able-bodied athlete, the dimension of difficulty, particularly with the swim and handcycle components, increases for the wheelchair triathlete. While the able-bodied triathlete spreads the length of a triathlon throughout a range of muscle groups, the wheelchair triathlete is restricted to arm and back muscles. Often a wheelchair triathlete—and Bailey is a good example of this—has no stomach muscles to use, an issue affecting power and balance. Unable to kick, the swim demands greater work from the upper body to provide rotation and counter drag. The equipment itself provides another set of problems. For one, the lightest handcycles can be in the range of 35 pounds ("We called them Lincoln Town cars," Jacobs says), twice the weight of a tri bike; and instead of being propelled by the largest muscle groups of the body, like quadriceps, hamstrings, gluteals, and core muscles, the handcycle is powered by the arms and back. The same is true for the wheelchair used in the run, although wheelchair racers can take better advantage of descents and flats than runners can (ascents are another deal). Finally, whatever stress an able-bodied triathlete attributes to air travel with a bike, imagine having to travel as wheelchair triathletes do: they need to get from their home, to the airport, to the hotel, and to the race with a handcycle, racing wheelchair, and regular wheelchair in tow. This collection of hurdles was the dramatic backdrop for Dr. Jon Franks, the first wheelchair triathlete to attempt the Hawaii Ironman in 1994. Franks didn't make the bike cut off, but he did complete the 112-mile leg on a handcycle.

After Franks, wheelchair triathlete John Maclean took up the goal. Jacobs suggested to Bailey they observe the 1997 Hawaii Ironman in person. "We went over on purpose," Jacobs says. "To watch MacLean, to see if it could be done." MacLean made the bike cut off and went on to successfully complete the race in the year the physically challenged division debuted. The fire was ignited in Bailey. "After the race, David wasn't home a week before he quit his job and started training. I think I got blamed for that one."

The qualifying event was in Lubbock, Texas, at the Buffalo Springs Lake Half Ironman in West Texas. Three Kona slots were up for grabs. It was a legitimate test. In 1998, race-day temperatures climbed to 114 degrees. Bailey raced not only to win a slot, but to be the first wheelchair triathlete across the line.

During the bike portion of the race, Bailey could look over his shoulder and see a competitor behind him, maintaining contact. "David hammered, trying to drop this guy," Jacobs says. "I remember saying to David from the road, 'Uh, he's still back there.'"

Early in the run, Bailey used a steep, long uphill to his advantage, Jacobs telling him that the man who got to the top of the hill first was going to win the race. Bailey charged it and used the fast decline to make what would be the deciding breakaway of the day, going on to win. Finishing second, the man who Bailey spent the day trying to shake, was Carlos Moleda. But second is second, and in the context of winning versus losing and the psychological momentum the former produces, Bailey had taken a big step toward establishing the win in Kona. In the metaphysics of dominating an opponent, Bailey had set the flow of energy and expectation to his advantage.

At the 1998 Hawaii Ironman, the spotlight was on Bailey. Not only was he a superstar from the motocross world, he was deeply connected to San Diego's pro triathlon culture. Moleda recalls being witness to this phenomenon: "He knew everybody."

In the race, it was not all the man from San Diego. Although Bailey led him out of the Kailua Bay, 1:17 to 1:22, Moleda biked nearly an hour faster, 7:46 to 8:42, and picked up even more time on the run. Finishing times: Moleda 11:25:55, Bailey 12:34:43.

"Carlos was gnarly," Jacobs says with awe, remembering the utter shock of the upset. "He made sure David understood he was gnarly. Bailey beat the shit out of him in Lubbock, but in Kona, Dave got whacked. It was a nice, thorough waxing. I told David, 'You didn't let this happen. It wasn't about you letting something happen. He did it. *He did it to you.*'"

During his years as a pro, Jacobs had seen this brand of competitive ferocity in the likes of Mark Allen and Dave Scott, athletes who didn't just want to win or even had to win. "They hated to lose and would do anything to make sure they didn't lose," Jacobs says. "And that was Carlos. Carlos was a former Navy SEAL, and a complete badass. He was someone who didn't seek out the cleanest lines, like David did, but who went right through the darkness. He didn't avoid fear; he went straight for it. I guess a day at Ironman isn't so bad once you've been shot at with machine guns.

"I said to David, 'Do you understand who it is you're messing with here? If you want to beat this guy, you're going to have to get bloody.'"

Getting beat was painful for Bailey. It harked back to his sentiment concerning the Ricky Johnson duel: "*It was the idea of someone being able to dominate me. I hated it.*"

* * *

Carlos Moleda was born in São Paulo, Brazil, in 1962, a year after David Bailey was born. A professional skateboarder in his teens who visited California in 1979, he decided at 18 to move to the United States. "My family thought I'd only last a month in the U.S., then turn around and come home," Moleda recalls.

Instead, Moleda would enlist in the U.S. Navy, securing his citizenship and volunteering to become a SEAL, arguably the most demanding of the armed forces' elite units. It was in SEAL training Moleda opened a door to the dark powers Jacobs refers to. "It was during the drown-proofing test, one of the tests you have to pass to qualify as a SEAL," Moleda explains. "They showed us what we were going to have to do. A lot of guys said, 'I'm out of here.'"

"After they tie your hands behind your back and your feet together, you jump into the deep end of a 50-meter pool. First you have to perform an underwater flip so that you're forced to start out with no momentum; no push off the wall or anything. You start from zero. Then you have to swim the length of the pool underwater, dolphin style."

On the weekend prior to the test, Moleda tried it out. He'd jump in, flip, and start swimming toward the other end. "Every time I tried, I'd get to about three-quarters of the way there and I'd have to come up for air." During the actual test, Moleda reached the point where he had been giving up. "I could see the wall. Right then, I made the decision I was going to make it." This time, Moleda touched the wall before coming up for air.

"I knew then what was possible when you reached deep for it," he adds. "I think everyone has the capacity for that kind of strength. They just don't know they have it. They haven't been put in a situation where they were forced to reach in and find it."

In December 1989, Moleda was a petty officer on SEAL Team Four when he was deployed in a mission to oust Manuel Noriega, the military dictator ruling Panama at the time. Among other things, the U.S. government wasn't keen about Noriega's spying on behalf of Cuba. Moleda's unit arrived in fast attack boats with the objective of disabling Noriega's Learjet. The unit received heavy fire—Moleda describes it as being in front of a firing squad—and a bullet lodged into his back. His legs went numb. He crawled through crossfire and was also shot in the leg. The team successfully blew up the jet and Noriega was apprehended. (Noriega was sentenced to 30 years in a federal prison in Miami on charges for cocaine trafficking and money laundering. After serving 18 years of the sentence, it is expected he will be extradited to France to serve more prison time.)

When Moleda woke up, he told the nurse he would return to duty in a week. He only realized the extent of his injuries when he heard her say, "They have sports programs for paraplegics."

The bulk of the next year would be spent in treatment and rehab. Whatever trauma he faced during this time, he made quick work of becoming an athlete again. In 1991 he made a statement when he pushed his wheelchair from Miami to his hometown of Virginia Beach, Virginia, a 1,200-mile trip.

After racing marathons, Moleda read about the attempt by Franks to finish Hawaii. He thought, "I can do that."

I can do that. Sarah Moleda, his wife (and a Hawaii Ironman finisher), has been witness to the unwavering intent Carlos brings to any goal he undertakes. "He's hyper-focused. On every single thing he does. Nothing or no one is going to get between him and the goal. If he says he's going to do something, he does it. Unless it's something he can't control, like his body."

Sarah describes how, for example, two years ago they decided to build their dream home in Hilton Head, South Carolina. "We physically built it ourselves. We used subcontractors for the framing and foundation, but pretty much everything else was on our own. If there was something we wanted but couldn't buy, Carlos designed it and made it. It took 18 months. There was no day off. We were here every single day. This is how Carlos is: 'Building this house is now our job. This is what we're going to do.' It can be frustrating. There are times I like to put things off; he's like 'let's do it yesterday.'"

Originally from Australia, Andrew Chafer, a landscaper, is one of Moleda's neighbors. He is also a triathlete and finisher of seven Ironmans. When word rounded through the community how the Moleda's were going to build the house on their own, Chafer says he heard people saying, "They're crazy. They'll never be able to do it." Chafer had been a friend and training partner of Moleda for years. "I told them, 'Just watch.'"

"One day I was in the backyard," Chafer says, "and I looked over and saw Carlos in his chair trying to plant a 300-pound palm tree. I said, 'Hey Carlos, can you use a hand?' He said, 'No, I got it.'"

Sarah says that her husband's sense of commitment and tenacity are on full display when it comes to his sport. "When he's going to start training for a race, he'll say, 'Monday is doomsday.' And when he starts training, that's it. That's what he's going to do every day until he makes his goal."

The first time Moleda started training for the Ironman, he pushed himself through a long ride to the point of physical breakdown. "He came back from the ride and his eyes were literally sunk into his head," Sarah says. "I tried to tell him he looked awful, that he looked like he was about to die. He finally admitted, 'Yeah, I don't feel too good.'"

"He's a crazy man," Chafer says. "He will go out on a seven-hour ride, purposefully forcing him to bonk."

Like many able-bodied triathletes, Moleda pinned his strategy on the 112-mile bike section of the race. "You have to focus on the bike," he says. "Don't worry about the swim or the run. The bike is the key." Using the old-school endurance training formula of *the more the body endures, the more it will endure,* Moleda has cranked his handcycle through all manner of pain and cramping, tempering his muscles to sustain a fast pace even when fatigued. According to

Sarah, Moleda has been advising his neighbor on how to properly prepare to take a shot at qualifying for the Hawaii Ironman, something Chafer has yet to accomplish. "He tells Andrew that he will need to go until he drops," Sarah reports. "It's okay if you don't finish the race. If your body craps out on you and you bomb, you will go away knowing you gave it your best shot and nothing less."

In 1999, this emphasis again catapulted Moleda to victory. Although Bailey swam 1:14 to Moleda's 1:17, he again got beat on the bike, 7:28 to 7:14. For the second year in a row, Bailey lost and had to suffer through the five-hour flight back to his home in San Diego.

"I wanted something bad," Bailey says. "But there was one other guy on the planet who wanted the same thing. His strength was that he always goes hard. He never played it safe. He beat me and I gave up. I was the better athlete, but he was the better man. Carlos ultimately made me better. There was always something more I could give, and he forced me to dig it up. I was like, 'Dammit. Why does this guy have to be so tough?' But looking back, I was grateful."

The drama before their 2000 rematch was heightened by Bailey's all-or-nothing commitment to it. He had decided that win or lose, 2000 would be his last Hawaii Ironman. Bailey's agonizing desire to win fueled the emotional urgency not only for him but also for Jacobs.

Jacobs believed the training and racing '99 and '00 were prerequisites for Bailey. "He needed the base from those two years to be able to do the kind of training he would need to beat Carlos. Carlos was like Steve Prefontaine. If you don't go with him when he goes off the front, he's going to beat you. You can't think that any amount of pacing will give you a chance. You can't hope he blows up. He will win. Carlos was willing to go hard early in the day and blast through his reserves. David was going to have to go with him."

On the psychological front, Jacobs spent many hours talking and training with Bailey. They would ride six and seven hours together at 17 to 18 mph. A great deal of soul searching occurred for both of them. For Bailey it was about giving his absolute all to a goal that, unlike motocross, he wasn't born to do; for Jacobs it was about coming to terms with professional regret.

"I consider my professional triathlon career a failure. In the years of working with David, I learned a great deal about myself and about sport, more than I did when I was actually a pro triathlete. The reason I didn't succeed when I was in it wasn't because I lacked talent or didn't work hard enough. It was about appreciation. It was about patience. I didn't enjoy it as much as I should have. I didn't understand what a gift it was. Ultimately I didn't have it mentally back then. These are things David has taught me."

Bailey took up the bonk-on-purpose training cry. "I checked out after the 1999 race. I ate doughnuts and got fat. But then I launched into the strictest regimen I'd ever been in." Bailey nailed a photo of Moleda to the wall. He'd heard that his competitor believed a 10:30 race in Kona was possible and was training for it. Bailey bolstered his training to prepare for the same target. After 40-mile rides he would tack on an additional five-mile time trial at 23 mph. Once on a long ride he rode straight into the deep cavern of a premium bonk. Desperate for fuel, he turned into a McDonald's drive through and ordered the works. Pulling into a parking space, in full view of the mystified diners inside wondering what this guy was doing in his space-age contraption handcycle, he spilled his Coke and fries onto the blacktop. He looked down at the mess, shrugged, and began feasting on them. Bailey's weekly training volume hit levels of 5,000 yards of swimming, 240 miles of cycling, and 90 miles in his racing wheelchair.

At times, the fierce workload would get to Bailey. "I would tell Todd how hard the training was and he'd say, 'David, this isn't hard. Hard is welding or driving a cab. Hard is trying to take care of a family of four on $35,000 a year. That's hard. Training, Dave, is awesome.'"

Reminiscent of the 1989 Ironwar, which pit a victory-starved Mark Allen against six-time winner Dave Scott, Bailey worked at replicating what Allen did to Scott: he locked on Moleda's tail and endeavored to stay there. Swim split: David Bailey 1:16:33, Moleda 1:16:32.

The pinnacle race of their series was held on a day in Hawaii that would go down as one of the windiest. Out of the water, Moleda used the handcycle to made a statement. "Carlos smoked me on the first hill," Bailey says. "Out on the highway, he was still getting away. I began thinking, 'No way can he go this fast all day.' And then the wind started hitting, and I swear, it didn't slow him down at all."

Bailey fought to keep contact and concentration. "It's a long race, and if you let your mind drift from the task, all of a sudden you've slowed down a mile or two per hour for 10 to 20 minutes."

Regardless, Moleda had established a huge gap. When Jacobs saw Moleda ride by after the Hawi turnaround, he didn't see Bailey for nearly seven minutes.

By his own account, Jacobs nearly lost it, screaming at Bailey when he came by to get back in it. *"This is your life right here! This is critical! This is everything! You have to pour everything into it! All of your disappointments, all of your pity, all of your anger, you have to lay it out right now!"*

In the ride back to Kona, Bailey clawed his way back into contact. Into T-2, after Bailey biked 7:26 to Moleda's 7:24:51, the race was going to come down to the marathon.

Once again, Moleda started off with a burst of speed. "I pounded as hard as I could," Moleda recalls. Bailey chose to focus on eating and drinking and not wasting energy going through town. Out of town and onto the Queen K again, Bailey began to push. At the turnoff into the Natural Energy Lab, Moleda held a 95-second lead.

For the first time in the three years of racing together, Bailey sensed Moleda was cracking. After the three miles of the Lab's out-and-back stretch, Bailey had caught up to Moleda. Bailey took a moment to fix his gloves and then attacked, flying by him. "The bear had jumped on my back," Moleda says. "After he passed me, he looked back. You could see it in his eyes: 'I got him.' His arms were just flailing. He was gone."

In the final stretch on Ali'i Drive, Bailey says he looked back over his shoulder again and again, terrified Moleda had resumed his supernatural-seeming abilities to snatch the victory from his hands. He didn't. When Bailey crossed the line, you could read his lips. He said, "Finally." Bailey's time was 11:05, 24 minutes faster than he raced in 1999.

"It was an honor for me to lose to him," Moleda says now, reflecting on the race. "He proved to everyone his grit. I dropped him on the bike. When I passed him I thought, 'He's gone.' But he was the better man."

"Those two gave as much as Dave and Mark did in '89," Jacobs says. "The race between them transcended the pro race that day. You hear about the sportsmanship between Carlos and David. Maybe outside of the race, but during it was personal. You have to make it personal in a combative sense. While the race is on, it's 'fuck you.'"

Bailey made good on his promise to leave Kona behind him, and has not returned. Although forever connected to the sport of triathlon, he is now an expert commentator for ESPN's motocross coverage. He has become a passionate advocate that riders use a protective brace—called a Leatt-Brace—to reduce the possibility of spinal cord injury (he makes a moving plea to riders in a YouTube video to make adopting the brace mandatory, the way seatbelts have been adopted in cars).

Moleda did return, in 2005, after struggling through complications following an accident on his chair requiring a series of surgeries and recoveries. Sitting down as much as paraplegics and quadriplegics do, pressure sores and infections are a constant threat, and potentially fatal. Moleda had three surgeries, each followed by more than half a year of recovery. "I got through it by telling myself that once it was all over, I would begin training again. I would spend my time thinking up training plans in my head."

Moleda's comeback, when you think about what he has survived to even attempt it, is the most stunning of his many accomplishments. Although bedridden for up to seven months after each of the surgeries, he recovered and began training. In 2005, tested by the talented and tough Marc Herremans, Moleda strung together a 1:17 swim, a 6:43 bike, and 2:23 run to do what he long ago believed was possible: 10:30. Now that the house is finished, Moleda has again begun training. Not for Kona, but for another goal, the Race Across America.

In addition to an assortment of causes the pair contributes to, Bailey and Moleda continue to work for the Challenged Athletes Foundation and other similar organizations. To learn more about the foundation and to see how you can help, visit www.ChallengedAthletes. org. Advancements in research indicate that the prospects of repairing spinal cord injuries are promising. For more information and a list of foundations, visit the National Institute of Neurological Disorders and Stroke website, NINDS.NIH.gov.

15
WHAT'S
NEXT?

MOVE UP TO THE OLYMPIC DISTANCE WITH COACH D'S TWELVE-WEEK PLAN

A triathlon freak since 1981, Duane Franks has also become a veteran multisport coach in the San Francisco Bay Area. I first met the 12-time Ironman finisher when the Golden Gate Triathlon Club (GGTC) was being formed in the early 1990s. Franks, who is also known as Coach D, always seemed to approach triathlon with the perfect balance of intellect and passion. He still does. Coach D continues to build on his legend as an age-group triathlete, but he also has the hard-science goods: He's USAT-certified, has earned Fitness Director credentials issued by the ACSM, and has a master's degree in exercise physiology. In addition to coaching a GGTC Ironman group, Franks operates his own coaching business, Trifiniti.

We asked Duane to construct a high-quality, simple-to-follow training program for the triathlete aspiring to move up to the challenge of an Olympic-distance race—a two-hour event for the pros, and three-plus hours for normal folk. Coach D delivered. After establishing the fitness and lifestyle you have at this point in the book, you're ready to push it to a new level.

And there's a cool side benefit: when the Olympics roll around every four years, you can compare your times to the world-class triathletes you're watching on TV.

A brief overview of Coach D's plan shows that the 12 weeks are grouped into three sets of four weeks. The goal of the first set is "aerobic endurance," which aims to slowly build your cardio. The second set of four-week training is to "build"—strengthen and speed up. The third and final set is to hone your speed and endurance to a peak that will leave you in top form for race day.

On a daily basis, for the most part, the midweek workouts mix all three sports of triathlon along with stretching and weight training. Generally, every Friday is a hard swim day, every Saturday is a long bike ride or a "brick" (a bike-run, bike-swim, or swim-run combo), every Sunday a long run, and every Monday a rest day. Every fourth week is recovery, with the 12th week leaving you rested and perfectly peaked for race day.

For more information on Coach D, go to his website (www.Trifiniti.com) or e-mail him at duane@trifiniti.com.

Week 1

Goal: Aerobic Endurance.

Monday: Swim easy and relaxed 800 yards/meters. Include drills (right arm/left arm/catch-up).

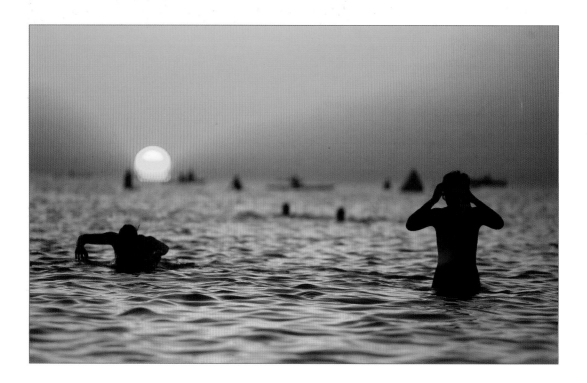

Tuesday: Run 20–30 minutes, easy to moderate effort. Focus on good rhythm. Do 10–20 minutes of stretching and core exercises. Strength train or yoga option.

Wednesday: Bike 30–45 minutes, easy to moderate effort. Focus on pedaling in circles instead of pushing up and down. Cadence of 85–95 rpm.

Thursday: Run 20–30 minutes, easy to moderate effort on flat to hilly terrain. 10–20 minutes of stretching and core exercises. Strength train or yoga option.

Friday: Swim 300 easy. Then swim 500 steady time trial. Then 200 easy. Total: 1000 yards/meters. Divide time trial time by 5 to calculate 100 base pace.

Saturday: Bike 60–90 minutes, easy to moderate effort on mostly flat to rolling terrain. Shift gears to keep a steady 85–95 cadence.

Sunday: Run 40–60 minutes, easy to moderate effort on flat to rolling terrain; if possible on dirt or other soft surface.

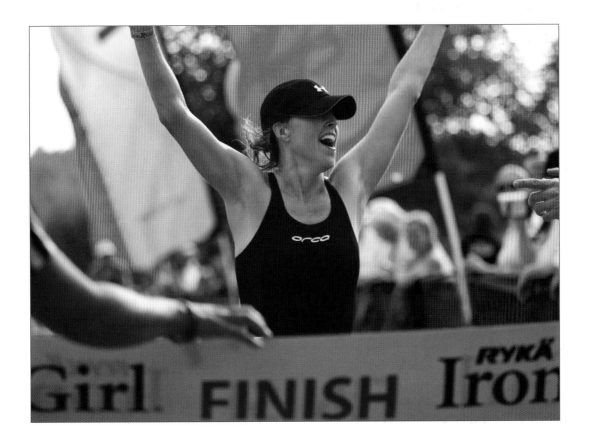

Week 2

Goal: Aerobic Endurance.

Monday: Complete rest day.

Tuesday: Run 25–35 minutes, moderate effort. Focus on good form and turnover. Do 10–20 minutes of stretching and core exercises. Strength train or yoga option.

Wednesday: Swim 200 easy. 300 with drills every other lap. 2 × 300s building to base pace. 100 easy cooldown. Total: 1200. Bike 40–60 minutes, easy to moderate effort. Include 10 minutes of higher than normal cadence.

Thursday: Run 25–35 minutes, easy to moderate effort on flat to hilly terrain. Lean forward, shorten stride, and use arms to lead the rhythm of the legs while climbing. Do 10–20 minutes of stretching and core exercises. Strength train or yoga option.

Friday: Swim 1300 pyramid intervals: 50, 100, 200, 300, 300, 200, 100, 50. Steady effort slightly slower than base pace. Allow 5–10 seconds rest between each interval.

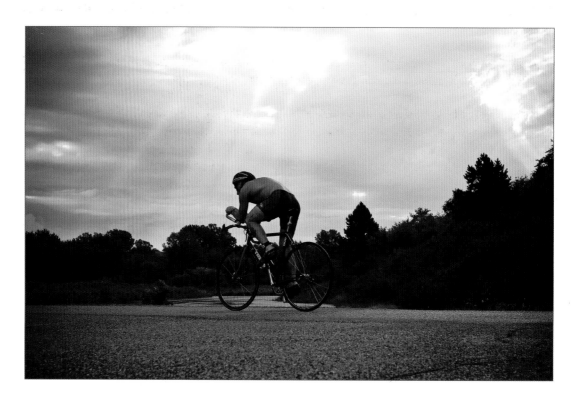

Saturday: Bike/run "brick": Bike 40–70 minutes, easy to moderate effort, followed by a quick transition and 15–25 minute run at easy to moderate effort. Reduce stride length and increase turnover to help transition into run.

Sunday: Run 45–60 minutes easy to moderate effort on flat to rolling terrain; if possible on dirt or other soft surface.

Week 3
Goal: Build.

Monday: Bike 30–45 minute easy spin at comfortably high cadence (90+ rpm).

Tuesday: Run 30–40 minutes at moderate effort. After warm-up, include 10–15 minutes at higher tempo (slightly slower than current 10K race pace). 10–20 minutes of stretching and core exercises. Strength train or yoga option.

Wednesday: Swim 300 easy. 100 kick with board. 5 × 100s at base pace with 10 seconds rest interval. 200 with alternate stroke (breast, back) on every other lap. 200 easy cooldown. Total: 1300. Bike 40–65 minutes, easy to moderate effort. Include 10 minutes of higher than normal cadence.

Thursday: Run 30–45 minutes, easy to moderate effort on flat to rolling terrain. Do 10–20 minutes of stretching and core exercises. Strength train or yoga option.

Friday: Swim 1500 in reverse ladder: 500, 400, 300, 200, 100. Allow 10 seconds rest between intervals. Goal is to increase pace as the interval becomes shorter. Final 100 easy cooldown.

Saturday: Bike 75–120 minutes, easy to moderate effort with rolling or hilly terrain. Stay seated while climbing. Focus on smooth and steady pedaling. Stay well hydrated.

Sunday: Run 50–65 minutes easy to moderate effort on rolling to hilly terrain; if possible on dirt or other soft surface.

Week 4
Goal: Recovery 1.

Monday: Complete rest day.

Tuesday: Run 20–30 minutes, easy effort. Focus on good running form and turnover. Do 10–20 minutes of stretching and core exercises. Strength train or yoga option.

Wednesday: Swim 200 easy. 6 × 75s (25 easy, 25 drill, 25 easy). Kick 4 × 50s with board. 200 easy cooldown. Total: 1050.

Thursday: Bike 30–45 minutes, easy recovery spin on mostly flat terrain. Comfortably high cadence. Focus on good pedaling technique, applying pressure on pedals throughout full 360 degrees.

Friday: Swim 1500 ladder: 100, 200, 300, 400, 500. Increase rest interval from 10 to 30 seconds as the intervals increase in length. Final 100 easy cooldown.

Saturday: Bike 60–90 minutes, easy ride on mostly flat to gently rolling terrain. Higher than normal cadence.

Sunday: Run 40–60 minutes, easy effort on mostly flat to rolling terrain; if possible on dirt or other soft surface.

Week 5

Goal: Build.

Monday: Bike 45–60 minutes, easy spin at comfortably high cadence (90+ rpm).

Tuesday: Run 35–45 minutes at moderate effort. After warm-up, include 15–20 minutes at higher effort tempo (slightly slower than 10K race pace). Do 10–20 minutes of stretching and core exercises. Strength train or yoga option.

Wednesday: Swim 300 easy. 8 × 50s (25 drill, 25 swim). 2 × 200s at base pace with 12 seconds rest between intervals. 200 easy cooldown. Total: 1300. Bike 40–65 minutes with 15–20 minutes at higher effort tempo. Stay in low aerodynamic position.

Thursday: Run 35–50 minutes easy to moderate effort on flat to rolling terrain. Do 10–20 minutes of stretching and core exercises. Strength train or yoga option.

Friday: Swim 1600 pyramid: 100, 200, 300, 400, 300, 200, 100. Goal is to swim the intervals on the backside faster than the front. Allow 10–15 seconds rest between intervals. Final 100 easy cooldown. OR swim approximately one mile in open water with wetsuit if you plan to race in a wetsuit. Steady, comfortable effort.

Saturday: Bike/run brick. Bike 50–90 minutes (or 75 percent of race distance) at moderate effort. Practice staying low on bars for good aerodynamics. Practice eating and drinking on bike. Prepare for quick transition to run. Run 20–30 minutes (or 66 percent of race distance) at moderate effort.

Sunday: Run 45–65 minutes. Begin easy then build to moderate effort during final 20–30 minutes.

Week 6

Goal: Build (race specific).

Monday: Complete rest day.

Tuesday: Run 40–50 minutes at moderate effort. After warm-up, include 5 × 3 minute intervals at approx 5K race effort. Three minute easy jog between. Balance is easy. Do 10–20 minutes of stretching and core exercises. Strength train or yoga option.

Wednesday: Swim 300 easy. 6 × 75s (25 alternate stroke, 25 drill, 25 easy). 6 × 100s at base pace with 10 seconds rest between intervals. 100 easy cooldown. Total: 1450. Bike 45–70 minutes with various hills. Build intensity as you reach the top of each hill. If no hills are available, select higher gears for 15–20 minutes of the ride.

Thursday: Run 35–50 minutes, easy to moderate effort on flat to rolling terrain. Do 10–20 minutes of stretching and core exercises. Strength train or yoga option.

Friday: Swim 500 time trial #2 to check progress and base pace. Repeat week 1 time trial. OR swim approximately one mile in open water with a wetsuit if you plan to race in a wetsuit. Steady, comfortable effort.

Saturday: Bike/run "brick": Bike 60–100 minutes (or 100 percent of race distance). Same as week 5. Prepare for quick transition to run. Run 25–40 minutes (or 75 percent of race distance) at moderate effort.

Sunday: Run 50–65 minutes (or 100 percent of race distance). Begin easy then build to moderate effort during final 20–30 minutes.

Week 7

Goal: Build—Overdistance.

Monday: Bike 45–60 minutes easy spin at comfortably high cadence (90+ rpm).

Tuesday: Run 40–50 minutes at moderate effort. After warm-up, include 6 × 3 minute intervals at 5K race effort. Three minute easy jog between. Balance is easy. Do 10–20 minutes of stretching and core exercises. Strength train or yoga option.

Wednesday: Swim 300 easy. 6 × 50s (25 drill, 25 swim). 2 × 200s at base pace with 15 seconds rest between intervals. 3 × 100s at base pace with 10 seconds rest between intervals. 100 easy cooldown. Total: 1400. Bike 40–65 minutes with 15–20 minutes at higher effort tempo. Stay in low aerodynamic position.

Thursday: Run 35–50 minutes, easy to moderate effort on flat to rolling terrain. Do 10–20 minutes of stretching and core exercises. Strength train or yoga option.

Friday: Swim double ladder: 100, 100, 200, 200, 300, 300, 400. Steady comfortable effort with only three to five seconds rest between intervals. 100 easy cooldown. Total: 1700.

Saturday: Bike 70–120 minutes (or 150 percent of race distance). Easy to moderate effort. Practice eating and drinking while riding.

Sunday: Run 60–75 minutes (or 110 percent of race distance). Steady, easy to moderate effort during final 20–30 minutes.

Week 8

Goal: Recovery.

Monday: Complete rest day. This will be a recovery week with less volume and intensity.

Tuesday: Run 20–30 minutes easy effort. Focus on good running form and turnover. Do 10–20 minutes of stretching and core exercises. Strength train or yoga option.

Wednesday: Swim 300 easy. 8 × 50s (25 drill, 25 easy). Pull 4 × 50 with buoy and paddles. 200 easy. Total: 1100.

Thursday: Bike 30–45 minutes, easy recovery spin on mostly flat terrain. Comfortably high cadence. Focus on good pedaling technique. Do 10–20 minutes of stretching and core exercises. Strength train or yoga option.

Friday: Swim 1550 pyramid: 50, 100, 150, 200, 250, 300, 200, 150, 100, 50. Steady relaxed effort. 5–10 seconds rest between intervals.

Saturday: Bike 60–90 minutes, easy on mostly flat to gently rolling terrain. Higher than normal cadence.

Sunday: Run 40–60 minutes, easy effort on mostly flat to rolling terrain; if possible on dirt of other soft surface.

Week 9

Goal: Build—Race specific.

Monday: Bike 45–60 minutes, easy spin at comfortably high cadence (90+ rpm).

Tuesday: Run 45–60 minutes at moderate effort. After warm-up, include 6 × 5 minute intervals at 10K race effort. Three minute easy jog between. Balance is easy. Do 10–20 minutes of stretching and core exercises. Strength train or yoga option.

Wednesday: Swim 300 easy. 4 × 50s (25 drill, 25 swim). 2 × 300s at base pace 20 seconds rest interval. 4 × 100s at base pace; 10 seconds rest between intervals. 100 easy cooldown. Total: 1600. Bike 40–65 minutes with 20–25 minutes at higher effort tempo. Stay in low aerodynamic position.

Thursday: Run 40–55 minutes, easy to moderate effort on flat to rolling terrain. Do 10–20 minutes of stretching and core exercises. Strength train or yoga option.

Friday: Complete rest day. Stretching and core exercises only. Practice pre-race dinner the night before. Plan how you will pack your transition bag. Practice placing race numbers on belt. Equip shoes with fast lace-locking system.

Saturday: Practice pre-race breakfast at least two hours before start of training. Swim/bike/run brick: Swim 100 percent of race distance, starting slow and building to what feels like race effort for the final 50 percent. Quick transition to bike and ride 100 percent of bike distance. Quick transition to run and run 20 minutes or 75 percent of run distance (whichever is longer). Maintain easy to moderate effort on bike and run. If possible, complete this workout on the actual racecourse. Practice race day nutrition and hydration.

Sunday: Run 60–75 minutes (or 110 percent of race distance). Build pace as you go. 20 minutes easy, 20 minutes moderate, 20 minutes fast. Balance is easy.

Week 10

Goal: Peak.

Monday: Complete rest day.

Tuesday: Run 45–65 minutes at moderate effort. After warm-up, include 7 × 3 minute intervals at 5K race effort. Three minutes easy jog between intervals. Balance is easy. Do 10–20 minutes of stretching and core exercises. Strength train or yoga option.

Wednesday: Swim 300 easy. 4 × 50s kick with board (fins optional). Pull 4 × 50s with buoy (paddles optional). 3 × 200s at base pace 20 seconds rest between intervals. 3 × 100s descending pace (100 easy, 100 moderate, 100 fast) with 10–12 seconds rest between intervals. 100 easy cooldown. Suggest using pull buoys (no paddles) for most of the swim to simulate wetsuit buoyancy. Total: 1700. Bike 40–65 minutes with 20–25 minutes at higher effort tempo. Stay in low aerodynamic position.

Thursday: Run 40–55 minutes, easy to moderate effort on flat to rolling terrain. Do 10–20 minutes of stretching and core exercises. Strength train or yoga option.

Friday: Swim 500 TT #3 to check progress and base pace. Repeat week 1 and 6 time trial. Add 300 extra to cooldown. Total: 1300.

Saturday: Swim/bike "brick": Swim 125 percent of race distance, starting slow and building to race effort during the final 50 percent. Quick transition to bike and ride 150 percent of race distance. Start easy then build to race effort for the final 20–30 minutes. Stay low on bars for good aerodynamics. Practice race day nutrition and hydration.

Sunday: Run 65–80 minutes (or 110 percent of race distance). Build pace as you go. 20 minutes easy, 20 minutes moderate, 20 minutes fast. Balance is easy.

Week 11

Goal: Peak.

Monday: Bike 45–60 minutes easy spin at comfortably high cadence (90+ rpm).

Tuesday: Run 45–60 minutes at moderate effort. After warm-up, include 6 × 6 minute intervals at 10K race effort. Three minute easy jog between. Balance is easy. Do 10-20 minutes of stretching and core exercises. Strength train or yoga option.

Wednesday: Swim 200 easy. 4 × 50s (25 drill, 25 swim). 2 × 300s at base pace with 20 seconds rest between intervals. 6 × 100s at base pace; 10 second rest interval. 100 easy cooldown. Suggest using pull buoys (no paddles) for most of the swim to simulate wetsuit buoyancy. Total: 1700. Bike 40–65 minutes with 25–40 minutes at race effort. Stay in low aerodynamic position.

Thursday: Run 40–55 minutes, easy to moderate effort on flat to rolling terrain. Do 10–20 minutes of stretching and core exercises. Strength train or yoga option.

Friday: Complete rest day. Stretching and core exercises only. Second opportunity to practice pre-race dinner the night before.

Saturday: Practice second pre-race breakfast at least two hours before start of training. Swim/bike/run brick: Swim 100 percent of race distance, starting slow and quickly building to what feels like race effort for the final 75 percent. Quick transition to bike and ride 75–100 percent of bike distance. Quick transition to run 15 minutes or 66 percent of race distance (whichever is longer). Maintain easy to moderate effort on bike and run. If possible, complete this workout on the actual racecourse. Practice race day nutrition and hydration.

Sunday: Run 55–65 minutes (or 100 percent of race distance). Build pace as you go. 10 minutes easy, 20 minutes moderate, 30 minutes fast. Balance is easy.

Week 12

Goal: Race taper.

Monday: Bike 30–45 minutes easy spin at comfortably high cadence (90+ rpm).

Tuesday: Run 30 minutes with 6 × 1-minute pick-ups at what feels like race effort. Allow two to three minutes between the intervals. Balance is easy. Do 10–20 minutes of stretching and core exercises. Strength train or yoga option.

Wednesday: Swim 200 easy. 2 × 150s (50 easy, 50 moderate, 50 fast). 20 seconds rest between intervals. 6 × 50s fast; 15 seconds rest interval between. Suggest using pull buoys (no paddles) for entire workout to simulate wetsuit buoyancy. Total: 800 yards. Bike 30–40 minutes. Include 6 × 1-minute pick-ups at race effort; allow two to three minutes between the intervals. Balance is easy.

Thursday: Rest day. Light stretching and core exercises only.

Friday: Bike 20–30 minutes easy effort. Shift through all gears to check mechanical performance. Stretch well after.

Saturday: Run 10 minutes easy. Include 5 × 30 sec pick-ups at race effort. Bike 10 minutes easy. Swim five to seven minutes easy. Open water with wetsuit if you plan to race in a wetsuit. Pre-race dinner as practiced.

Sunday: Race day! Pre-race breakfast as practiced. Sprint or Olympic Triathlon. Pace as you practiced. Good Luck!

INTENSITY TERMS

Easy Effort: This is active recovery, approximately 50–67 percent of maximum heart rate.

Moderate Effort: This is aerobic endurance, approximately 68–79 percent of maximum heart rate.

Higher Effort: This is approximate lactate threshold or sustained race pace, 80–89 percent of maximum heart rate.

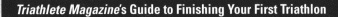
Coach D's Tips:

1. Have a knowledgeable swimmer or coach evaluate your swim stroke and prescribe specific drills to help optimize efficiency. It's easier to establish proper stroke mechanics when first learning. Poor stroke habits are hard to break.

2. The key to improving fitness is to progressively build duration and intensity. However, our body absorbs the training and adapts by getting stronger during rest. Recovery workouts and complete rest are required to get faster. Include a recovery week every fourth week.

3. Master athletes over age 40 should consider resting more often than younger athletes. Athletes over age 50 should schedule a full recovery week every second or third week.

4. Include stretching and core exercises two to three times a week. Swimming, cycling, and running for long durations require a strong core and flexibility.

5. Strength training during the build and peak phase should be limited to maintenance and triathlon-specific exercises. Consult a triathlon coach or personal trainer for help designing a strength program to compliment your endurance training.

6. Run on dirt or another soft surface whenever possible. Running on asphalt and especially concrete results in greater musculoskeletal impact and can lead to injury.

7. Adjust your caloric intake to match expenditure. Endurance training requires energy to perform workouts. If you're trying to lose weight, create a caloric deficit (difference between intake and expenditure) of no more than 500 calories a day. This will result in approximately one pound of weight loss per week. A nutrition expert can analyze your diet and help plan healthy meals.

8. Stay well hydrated by drinking before, during, and after exercise. Monitoring your body weight will help you replace lost fluids. Drink one pint of water for every pound lost.

9. Include mental training. A good sports psychologist can help you develop strategies and tools to gain the mental edge needed for times when training becomes physically and emotionally challenging.

10. Identify goals for training and racing. Training goals should be specific and measurable and should support your race goals. Keep it fun. Remember the reason you entered the race. Sometimes the process is the goal, so enjoy the journey.